Opposites Attract

How to Use the Secrets of Personality Type
to Create a Love That Lasts

Renee Baron

Illustrations by Anne Gibbons

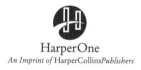

HarperOne
An Imprint of HarperCollinsPublishers

This book is dedicated to my family and friends
with love and gratitude

HarperOne

Appendices A and B adapted from *What Type Am I?* by Renee Baron, copyright © 1998 by Renee Baron. Used by permission of Penguin, a division of Penguin Group (USA) Inc.

MBTI, Myers-Briggs, and *Myers-Briggs Type Indicator* are registered trademarks of the MBTI Trust, Inc.

FIRST EDITION

Library of Congress Cataloging-in-Publication Data
is available upon request.

ISBN 978–0–06–191429–4

Illustrations © 2011 by Anne Gibbons

11 12 13 14 15 RRD(H) 10 9 8 7 6 5 4 3 2 1

Contents

1

Welcome to the World of Opposites

Does it frustrate you that your quiet, reserved spouse never wants to have people over and you love socializing and entertaining?

Do you consider your partner to be rigid and uptight because she nags you about your messy office?

Are you fond of schedules and routines, but your casual and spontaneous boyfriend wants to just go with the flow and see whatever turns up?

Do you think of yourself as the arty, creative type, yet the love of your life is Mr. (or Ms.) Good Common Sense?

If so—welcome to the club!

In our relationships, especially our intimate ones, we often are attracted to people who are different from us. We seem to have an instinctive need to search for some "missing" part of ourselves in another person, whom we then depend on to supply the qualities that we lack or have not yet developed. The reserved person, for example, may depend on a mate who is outgoing and gregarious to provide a social circle, and the talkative, outgoing type may crave a partner who won't compete with him for attention.

In the beginning these differences are positive, intriguing, even dazzling. We think that we've found the perfect match. And then a little time goes by. The infatuation fades, the newness wears off, the honeymoon is over—and all that was appealing before starts to become downright irritating.

Perhaps your partner, whose levelheadedness and rationality you once admired and appreciated for balancing out your flighty, emotional personality, now drives you crazy with his coldness. Instead of lending a sympathetic ear when you have a problem, he quickly offers advice about how you should fix it. Meanwhile, he doesn't understand why you take remarks so personally and why your feelings are always getting hurt.

Perhaps, at first, your partner's ability to converse with many people was inspiring and invigorating. Now her chatter drives you up the wall, and you wish she could keep some of her thoughts to herself. You like a lot of solitude and time to yourself, and it's bothersome to be dragged to social events every weekend. Her need for interaction versus your need for solitude is driving the two of you apart.

Or maybe your spouse is that open-ended, go-with-the-flow person who always wants to change plans at the last minute, and you like having things settled and decided. He drags his heels, procrastinates, is always running at least half an hour late, and wonders why you can't seem to relax and let go once in a while.

> Men are from Earth. Women are
> from Earth. Deal with it.
>
> GEORGE CARLIN

Psychologists have many theories about why people can have such a hard time finding and sustaining healthy and satisfying relationships. We are often taught that gender is to blame; men and women are fundamentally different, according to this theory, and it has even been said, metaphorically, that they come from different planets. Although it's true that some women fit the stereotype of being sensitive,

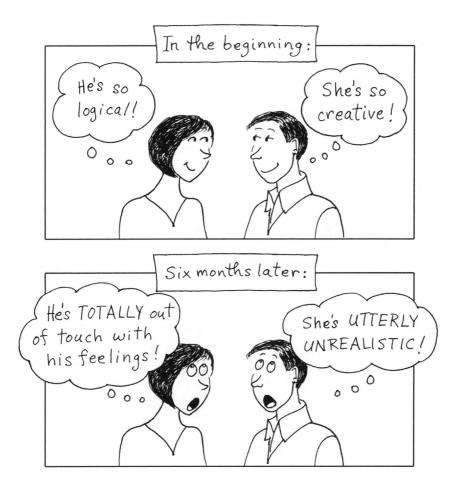

tenderhearted, and emotional, just as some men fit the stereotype of being logical, analytical, and emotionally self-contained, studies demonstrate that such men and women represent less than half of the population. Theories based on gender may benefit some of us, but they are not particularly useful to the majority of the population whose personalities do not conform to the stereotypes.

So if gender doesn't entirely account for the difficulties and conflicts we encounter as we try to maintain satisfying relationships, what does? Forty years ago, I was introduced to the concept of personality preferences in a workshop on the Myers-Briggs Type Indicator (MBTI®) inventory. I was both fascinated and astounded by this theory of human differences, which appeared to answer many long-held questions as to why people have such a hard time in their relationships—not only their intimate partnerships but their relationships with their children, siblings, co-workers, and friends. My study of the MBTI system over many decades, combined with my eyewitness perspective as a marriage and family therapist during that time, has led me to believe that personality preferences account for a great deal of what goes on between human beings.

A Brief History

The concept of personality preferences was originally developed by Carl Jung, the prominent Swiss psychoanalyst, and set forth in his well-known book *Psychological Types*, published in English in 1923. One reader profoundly affected by Jung's concept was an American woman, Katharine Briggs, an astute student of human nature who had already spent some years in an independent study of personality preferences and had developed her own typology. Recognizing that Jung's theory went far beyond her own, Briggs recruited her Swarthmore-educated daughter, Isabel Myers, to collaborate with her in studying and expanding the theory even further. Their aim was to help people better understand themselves and others by determining their personality types.

During the 1940s, Briggs and Myers created the first version of the now-famous questionnaire that measures inherent and observable differences in human behavior—that is, personality types. Over the years the mother-daughter team refined the questionnaire through diligent research. When Consulting Psychologists Press (CPP) took over the publication of the questionnaire in 1975, it became readily available for use by psychologists, career counselors, others in the helping professions, and those simply seeking a deeper understanding of themselves. Today the MBTI inventory, taken by two million people each year, is the most widely used and respected personality assessment instrument in the world.

In creating the MBTI inventory, Myers and Briggs had two goals in mind. The first was to allow respondents to identify their basic preference on each of four dimensions: (1) what energizes them, (2) how they experience the world, (3) how they make decisions, and (4) how they conduct their outer lives. Their second goal was to identify and describe each of the sixteen personality types that result from the interactions among the basic preferences. For the sake of clarity, this book focuses only on the first goal—identifying the preferences—which is the key to understanding the MBTI inventory.*

Personality Preferences

The inventory is composed of four sets of opposite personality preferences—extraverting versus introverting, sensing versus intuiting, thinking versus feeling, and judging versus perceiving. Please note that the MBTI inventory describes the preferences as adjectives but that, for the sake of simplicity, I use them as nouns—Extravert-Introvert, Sensor-Intuitive, Thinker-Feeler, and Judger-Perceiver. It's important, however, to keep the adjectival sense of each word in mind. For example, describing yourself as an introvert is a shorthand way of saying that you lean toward the introverting side of the scale, that you *prefer* introversion over extraversion.

These personality preferences describe different patterns of behavior that affect and determine how we function and act in the world. Differences in preferences have a profound impact on every aspect of our lives—from the way we get our energy to how we see the world and focus our attention, to how we make decisions, to how we like to live our daily lives.

1. **The Energizing Preference: Extraverting-Introverting**
    This preference relates to where we focus our attention and what energizes us.

    *   Extraverts† focus their attention outward and draw energy from the external world of people and things.

---

* For those who are interested, I offer a brief explanation of the sixteen types in Appendix A. This aspect of the MBTI is also covered in great detail in my book *What Type Am I?* (New York: Penguin, 1998).

† No, you haven't found a typo: "extraverting" may look strange, but the MBTI inventory uses this spelling, which is derived from German (the language in which Jung wrote).

- Introverts focus their attention inward and draw energy from their own inner world of thoughts and insights.

2. **The Perceiving Preference: Sensing-Intuiting**
   This preference relates to how we experience the world and take in information.

   - Sensors perceive the world through information absorbed from their five senses in the present moment. They focus on here-and-now reality.

   - Intuitives perceive the world through abstraction and imagination. They focus their attention on the future and on possibilities.

3. **The Decision-Making Preference: Thinking-Feeling**
   This preference relates to how we evaluate information and make decisions.

   - Thinkers make objective or impersonal decisions based on logic and analysis.

   - Feelers make decisions based on what is important to them and others personally, according to their subjective values.

4. **The Lifestyle Preference: Judging-Perceiving**
   This preference relates to how we shape our outer lives.

   - Judgers like closure and want to have things settled and decided as soon as possible.

   - Perceivers like to keep their options open.

In the context of the MBTI inventory, the word "preference" simply refers to how we naturally prefer to do things. A preference is a tendency to be, act, or think in a certain way. Preferences are similar to handedness. Everyone has both a right hand and a left hand, but most people "prefer" one over the other. Writing with the hand that we use every day is effortless, and we don't even think about it. Writing with our other hand, however, takes more time and requires more concentration; it feels awkward and our execution is less skillful.

It is also important to acknowledge that we all have aspects of both preferences. We couldn't function too well in the world if we didn't. But when we are acting in a way that is in keeping with our natural preference, we feel more confident, more competent, and pleasantly energized. Because we tend to be more at ease when we're functioning within our preference, we're more comfortable and successful as well.

Although different situations may temporarily draw us toward our opposite preference, our core preference remains constant throughout our lives. In other words, an Extravert never becomes an Introvert, and an Introvert never becomes an Extravert; a Thinker never becomes a Feeler, and a Feeler never becomes a Thinker; and so on. Nevertheless, we can develop our opposite preference more fully over time and become more at ease operating within it, especially in the latter part of life. For example, an Introvert may have always dreaded speaking in front of people, but his job responsibilities have helped him develop into a very confident speaker. Or a relatively disorganized person may discover her ability to stay on top of things when she becomes a caretaker for an elderly person.

These four sets of personality preferences do not, however, tell the whole story.

While everyone has a preference for one side of the axis or the other, we must also take into account the strength or degree of that preference. Each personality preference is not an absolute, but a point on a continuum. For example, maybe you are a strong Thinker (scoring high on the thinking continuum), while your spouse is also a Thinker, but with a less pronounced tendency.

Keep in Mind That . . .

- All preferences are equally valuable. No one preference is better than any other. There are no negative descriptions and no "bad" personality types. Each preference is associated with many potential strengths and some weaknesses.

- We can and do use all eight preferences many times every day, but we prefer to use our four favorites because they feel more natural and comfortable.

- Preferences are not indicators of ability, skill, or intelligence. Each preference indicates what we *like* to do, not what we *can* do.

- While we change and grow throughout our lives, our preferences stay the same. However, the strength of our preferences may vary considerably at different times, based on what our life experiences bring out in us and what we choose to bring out in ourselves.

Understanding preferences provides powerful yet practical insights into human behavior that can benefit us in our relationships with others and as individuals. On a personal level, knowing that our preferences are a core part of who we are can help us to be more accepting of ourselves. We tend to feel less guilty or judgmental about aspects of ourselves that we previously considered to be shortcomings. Through studying personality preferences, we begin to see that there is a good reason why we can't do everything in life equally well and that we do not have to struggle to be what we are not. We can also decide more easily which work environments and careers are best suited to our nature. We can even hope to begin to take ourselves less seriously and maybe even have a few good laughs in the process.

> One loses so many laughs by
> not laughing at oneself.
>
> SARA JEANNETTE DUNCAN

Preferences can also help us gain insights into human behavior that benefit us in our relationships. Developing a greater understanding of others leads to a more accepting attitude toward our romantic partner and lessens our inclination to try to change that person. We are more likely to see other people's behavior as simply *different* from our own, not as bad or wrong. And as we discover which people we naturally get along with and which ones are more likely to push our buttons, we gather useful information for assessing not only the probable success of our love relationships but the success of every other type of relationship in our lives as well.

I hope that learning about personality preferences deepens your understanding and appreciation of yourself and helps you honor and develop the strengths and abilities you bring to all of your relationships. I also hope that you become better able to see others' differences with more compassion and humor. When you are irritated with your partner, I hope that this understanding will give you a greater sense of detachment and help you see that your partner's behavior stems from a natural predisposition and not from a desire to make life difficult for you.

> Everything that irritates us about others can
> lead us to an understanding of ourselves.
>
> CARL JUNG

Learning about personality preferences can give you and your partner a common language so that you can communicate more effectively. Even though learning about personality preferences solves only one piece of the complex puzzle of relationships, it's an important piece, and one that can help you navigate all of your relationships toward a place of peace and understanding. I hope that this book provides you with a practical guide to arriving there.

2

Discover Your Preferences

The ten questions at the beginning of each chapter (sometimes also referred to as an inventory) will help you identify your preferences.* For each question, check the response that fits best—A or B.

You may identify somewhat with both statements in a pair, but one answer usually comes more easily, while its opposite seems less familiar to you. It's best not to think too long about the statements—go with your first, most automatic response. Remember, the inventories are designed only to help you find out more about yourself; they are not tests, and there is no "better" or "right" answer to any question. So do your best to respond based on what is really true for you rather than on what you think should be true.

At the end of the ten questions, in the first blank space, record how many times you chose A as the answer. In the second blank space, record how many times you chose B.

The higher your score on an inventory, the stronger your preference. If you come out somewhere in the middle, you may resonate with both sets of preferences, but only one will be your best fit.

10—A very strong preference

8 or 9—A medium-strong preference

6 or 7—A moderate preference

---

*Please note that my questions are not intended to take the place of the official MBTI, which is a much longer and more involved questionnaire and can be given only by someone who is certified to administer it and interpret the results.

5—Balanced in the middle, but you are likely to resonate with one more than the other when you read the chapter describing the two preferences.

It's more common to wind up with some A answers and some B answers than it is to wind up with a 10–0 (or 0–10) split. If you do come out with a significantly higher score on one than another—for example, 9 on Extravert and 1 on Introvert, or vice versa—you most likely have found your true preference. If your tendencies are more moderate, you will relate to some degree to both the Extravert and the Introvert preferences. However, it is common to have at least a slight preference for one over the other. If, for example, you wrote 6 next to Extravert and 4 next to Introvert, then Extravert is probably your stronger preference. If one side of a preference pair sounds about 60 to 70 percent like you, that is probably your favored preference. If you wrote 5 next to Extravert and 5 next to Introvert, you may want to check the inventory again. Your preferences one way or the other, however slight, will become clearer when you read each chapter and learn more about each preference.

Do keep in mind that the goal of the inventory is to help you find your *preferences,* not to provide labels. So a 10 on the line next to Extravert, for example, means that you *prefer* extraversion, or are more comfortable with it—not that you *are* an Extravert.

Those with a high score on one preference—a 9 or a 10, say—are often surprised at how closely my written description matches their way of being. Keep in mind, however, that you won't usually recognize yourself in every word about your preference. For clarity and humor, I tend to go to extremes in describing each of the types; most of us are not as intensely polarized as the examples presented here. Also, those with more moderate tendencies often relate to both preferences in a pair.

In any event, no matter how you score on the inventories, the degree to which you resonate with the descriptions in each chapter is most telling. If you decide that you have a preference for thinking over feeling, nobody is going to say otherwise—you, and only you, are in the best position to know.

Finding Your True Preference

Some people initially have difficulty finding their true preference on certain inventories. If this is the case for you, one of the following reasons probably explains your confusion.

- Feeling as though you should come across in a certain way may be making it difficult for you to separate your own experience from the expectations of others. You may have felt pressured by your family or by the society you grew up in to behave in ways that were not true to your natural self. For example, in the United States the Extravert preference is the accepted style of behavior. Introverts often feel that they should be more outgoing and sociable.

- Gender role expectations put pressure on men to appear logical, rational, and analytical and on women to appear warm, nurturing, and supportive. A conflict between expectation and reality can cloud the results of your inventory.

- If your work requires skills that don't utilize your natural preferences, you might find yourself answering in your "work mode" rather than according to your true preference. For example, you are perfectly capable of being as organized and structured in your way of thinking as your position requires, but this mode of being is nonetheless stressful and less preferable for you.

- The two people in some intimate relationships share many of the same preferences. If so, you may find yourself using one of your opposite preferences to bring balance to the relationship. For instance, when two Introverts are involved with each other, one will sometimes behave more like an Extravert and adopt a more outgoing role. Such switchovers can help couples function better, both in their intimate life and in the outside world.

- You may have entered a stage of your life when it's appropriate to develop your opposite preferences. At midlife many people open up to the less-developed parts of themselves. Also, at times of crisis or when your circumstances shift, such as after a divorce, a move, or a death, you may wish to change or reinvent yourself and try out new behaviors or activities.

- You might answer certain questions differently at different times depending on your mood, influential events, or other factors. If you are on the fence about a question, choose the answer that, over the long term, has most frequently been true for you.

If you continue to have difficulty identifying some of your preferences, you will probably gain clarity by keeping track of your behavior for a few weeks. Observe yourself and notice your choices, your natural inclinations, and your comfort level in different situations. Also, be sure to take your time reading each of the chapters; allow the process of self-observation and self-discovery to unfold at a natural pace. Each preference is rich in its own way, and the identification of your preferences can answer many important questions about yourself and your relationships with others.

How to Use This Book

Each of the four sections on the four sets of preferences begins with an inventory for you to complete and a brief description of both preferences. A dedicated description of each preference follows, along with suggestions for (1) acknowledging and appreciating your own type and (2) recognizing the type-based attitudes and behaviors that make it difficult for you to relate to someone of an opposing preference. A separate chapter focuses on practical relationship issues, explaining the typical dynamics between both couples of opposite preferences and same-preference pairs and providing time-tested tips for getting along better with your partner.

Ideally, both you and your partner will read the book and work together to complete the exercises for enhancing your relationship. Any relationship can be improved, however, even when only one member of the couple becomes more aware of his or her counterproductive behavior. Changing just one negative pattern can have a positive effect on your relationship as a whole. Whether you're embarking on this exploration alone or with your partner, I know you'll find the journey challenging at times (it takes courage to look closely at your own behavior), but also self-affirming and rewarding.

3

The Energizing Preference

EXTRAVERTS/INTROVERTS

Read the following statements and check the sentence that describes you best—A or B. To achieve the most accurate score, answer the statements according to what is true for you, not according to what you would like to be true or think ought to be true.

The Inventory*

1. A ☐ I feel energized when I interact with people.
   B ☒ I feel drained if I spend too much time with others.

2. A ☐ People would probably describe me as friendly or outgoing.
   B ☒ People would probably describe me as reserved or aloof.

3. A ☐ I prefer to develop ideas by discussing them with others.
   B ☒ I prefer to develop ideas by reflecting on them in my mind.

4. A ☐ I often enjoy being the center of attention.
   B ☒ I usually avoid being the center of attention.

---

* The following inventory is not associated with, nor does it represent or replicate, the authentic Myers-Briggs Type Indicator® instrument and its results. For the genuine MBTI® instrument, go to www.mbticomplete.com.

5. A ☐ I tend to say the first thing that comes into my mind, without thinking too much beforehand.

    B ☒ Before I speak, I usually consider what I'm going to say.

6. A ☐ I enjoy having a wide circle of friends and acquaintances.

    B ☒ I enjoy having just a few close friends.

7. A ☐ I tend to be talkative in groups.

    B ☒ I tend to be quiet in groups.

8. A ☐ When I spend long periods of time by myself, I can end up feeling lonely and restless.

    B ☒ I am comfortable spending a great deal of time alone.

9. A ☒ I prefer a job that involves working with ~~many~~ other people.

    B ☐ I prefer a job that allows me to work alone.

10. A ☐ I find it stimulating to socialize with a group of people.

    B ☒ I feel most comfortable socializing with just one or two other people at a time.

Scoring

In the first blank space below, record how many times you chose A as the answer to one of these ten questions. In the second blank space below, record how many times you chose B.

Total

__1__ A Extravert
__9__ B Introvert

Extraverts and Introverts in a Nutshell

Most of us would say that we are familiar with the terms "extravert" and "introvert." Asked for definitions, we would explain that the Extravert is outgoing and talkative, while the Introvert is shy and withdrawn—end of story. In the context of the MBTI instrument, however, many terms have very precise definitions that differ from how they are commonly used. That is certainly the case with this first set of preferences. Extraversion and introversion are thought of as referring to how people become energized and where they focus their attention. The key distinction between the two is whether energy and attention are directed outward or inward.

Extraverts mainly focus on the external world and experience an increase in energy and an enhanced sense of well-being when they interact with people, things, and activities outside of themselves. That's what keeps their batteries charged, so to speak. A high extraversion score means that almost everything you do relates primarily to the outer world. It does not mean that you are loud or boisterous.

Introverts mainly focus on their inner world and experience an increase in energy and an enhanced sense of well-being when they spend time contemplating their own ideas, impressions, thoughts, and feelings. Solitude and quiet are necessary for Introverts to recharge their batteries; otherwise, they feel ungrounded and out of sorts. A high introversion score means that you usually think things through by yourself before you act or respond and that you need a lot of time alone. It does not mean that you are quiet and withdrawn or at risk of becoming a hermit.

> Extraverts . . . cannot understand life until they have lived it. Introverts . . . cannot live life until they understand it.
>
> ISABEL BRIGGS MYERS

Every human psyche encompasses elements of extraversion and elements of introversion. On the deepest level, we don't change: Extraverts remain Extraverts, and Introverts remain Introverts. As Extraverts mature, however, they may learn to use their introverted side when it serves them, and Introverts may learn to use their extraverted side. The potential to move between preferences in this way, as noted in the introduction, applies to all four sets of opposite styles.

For those who are very strongly oriented toward extraversion, it can be quite uncomfortable to engage in introverted activities, and common consequences are restlessness, boredom, irritability, or moodiness. For others, the pull toward extraversion is not as strong; these Extraverts are capable of engaging in introverted activities (such as, but certainly not limited to, reading, writing, and solitary thinking) without experiencing too much stress. On occasion, they may even enjoy these pursuits, and at those times they can strongly resemble Introverts.

The same principles apply to Introverts. For those who are strongly oriented toward this preference, it can be quite uncomfortable to engage in extraverted activities. Spending too much time with others results in exhaustion and a desperate desire for solitude to reinvigorate the spirit. For other Introverts, the pull is not particularly strong, and they can spend longer periods of time with people without exhausting their reserves. Introverts of this type genuinely enjoy some extraverted activities and can even appear, for all practical purposes, to be Extraverts. But they are still Introverts.

Shattering Some Stereotypes

A common misperception is that a tendency toward extraversion or introversion is related to gender. Women, according to this stereotype, are Extraverts—strongly oriented toward social interaction, they prefer to talk things through rather than contemplate them alone and are uninhibited about seeking help from or contact with others. On the other hand, men, in this mistaken belief, are mostly Introverts— strong silent types, loners who have to do everything for themselves.

Another mistaken idea is that extraversion is somehow superior to introversion. If you think about it for a moment, you'll realize that different cultures value different personality traits. People in many Western cultures seem to be more comfortable with extraverted behavior—and nowhere more so than in the United States. In fact, 75 percent of the U.S. population are Extraverts, while only 25 percent are Introverts. In this country, we tend to interpret the Introvert's quiet ways and preference for solitude as antisocial and therefore as evidence of a character flaw that must be overcome. To avoid being judged in a negative manner, many Introverts in the United States learn to mimic extraverted behavior. Although some "perform" quite well in this mode, their underlying preference does not change, and the Introvert masquerading as an Extravert eventually suffers from—and resents—the need to present a false self.

Solitude is un-American.

ERICA JONG

Yet another false assumption is that all Introverts are shy and all Extraverts are socially confident. Shyness is a form of anxiety that leads us to avoid contact with others for fear of being rejected or ridiculed. Thus, both the shy and the introverted tend to shrink from social situations. But Introverts are not necessarily intimidated by other people—by nature, they're just not inclined to seek them out or to strike up conversations merely for the sake of human connection. A shy person, on the other hand, is not just inclined to avoid certain types of interpersonal interactions, but strongly motivated to do so. All this is not to say, of course, that some Introverts are not indeed shy, but it's important to realize that some other Introverts may be quite socially confident. Along the same lines, Extraverts may suffer from shyness—even more acutely, in some cases, than Introverts, since anxiety prevents them from fulfilling their deep underlying desire for social connection. As you continue to read, you'll see these stereotypes about Extraverts and Introverts for what they are—broad generalizations that may or may not apply to any given individual.

You Might Be an Extravert If . . .

- You invited one hundred of your closest friends to your fortieth birthday party.

- Standing in line at the grocery store becomes a social event.

- "The more the merrier" is one of the tenets you live by.

- You'd enjoy going on a week's vacation with a group of people who wouldn't let you have time to yourself except in the bathroom.

- "I'm speechless" is not part of your vocabulary.

- Your cell phone is listed in the company directory.

- You like being selected by the speaker as a volunteer to get up in front of the audience.

- Silence may be golden, but frankly, it makes you nervous.

- You have more Facebook friends than bytes of memory on your hard drive.

Extraverts at Their Best	Extraverts at Their Worst
Outgoing	Tactless
Energetic	Loud
Enthusiastic	Attention-seeking
Lively	Unable to be alone
Friendly	Restless
Sociable	Don't think before speaking
Initiating	Overly talkative
Upbeat	Dominate in conversations

Extraverts 101

I believe in the discipline
of silence and could talk for
hours about it.

GEORGE BERNARD SHAW

For an Extravert, interacting with others is the supreme energizer. Unlike inward-looking Introverts, Extraverts focus their attention externally—on things, people, and activities. They are more comfortable being with others than being alone. When solitary for too long, they become restless, lonely, or bored. You'll rarely find an Extravert hiking all alone in the wilderness with only the trees for company, although for many Introverts that would qualify as paradise. With other people around, as in a busy downtown district or a crowded café, an Extravert can tolerate—even enjoy—being alone . . . but only for a while.

Solitude is more enjoyable
when you have someone to
talk about it with.

ANONYMOUS

Immediately after work, the Extravert may crave a little time alone to unwind. But enough is enough. The second the Extravert catches sight of friends walking into the yoga class or goes to happy hour, those batteries start recharging, and along comes the proverbial second wind.

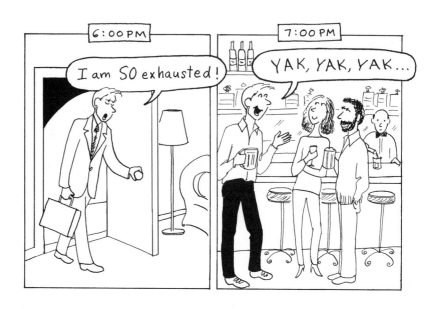

Social Life

Extraverts usually have a wide circle of friends and acquaintances and enjoy making plans with others. Typically, they engage in many activities, and their calendar is full of events and get-togethers.

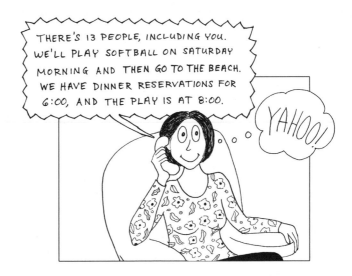

Playing host is a pleasure for many Extraverts, and their homes are frequently the center of buzzing social activity. A strong Extravert wouldn't dream of missing a birthday celebration, a good-bye party, or just the weekly lunch with a friend, although this extreme sociability may diminish somewhat with age. Committing themselves to too many activities can leave Extraverts feeling stressed. They can also become so busy that they neglect their loved ones.

At social gatherings, Extraverts like to circulate and interact with many people. Sticking with any one person or group for too long is draining to them, unless the conversation is extremely engaging. Strong Extraverts have a rather short attention span. Because they are constantly scanning the environment in order to see everything, they are easily distracted. If they are speaking with someone and then hear someone else talking about an interesting topic, as fascinating as their current conversation may be, they'll find a way to terminate it and move on.

Extraverts find new situations and people exciting and stimulating. When waiting in line at the movies or the supermarket, they are the ones who can strike up a conversation with a complete stranger. They can find a way to start talking to anyone who looks interesting. And if you ask them how they're doing, they'll tell you. Extraverts are usually easier to get to know than Introverts because they let you see more of who they are right away.

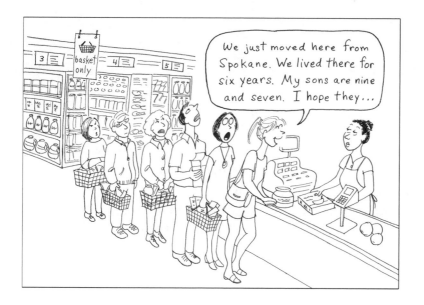

When it comes to dating, Extraverts have it easier than Introverts because of their relative ease in approaching and engaging with new people. They are able to make themselves known to a wider circle of people, so they meet potential mates more easily.

Extraverts' need to interact with others may evoke jealousy in a partner. Their friendliness can be seen as seductive, but often it's just a reflection of their outgoing style. Extraverts don't necessarily find marital fidelity challenging, but they can't stand to have their social life curtailed. An insecure partner will sometimes attempt to set limits on who the Extravert can associate with and under what circumstances. This strategy tends to backfire. Chances are that the cute neighbor or charismatic yoga teacher is no threat to the relationship—but having to rein in his or her natural impulse to be friendly can make an Extravert edgy enough to jump ship.

Communicating with an Extravert

> I can go on forever. To me, one thought
> becomes five hundred sentences.
>
> ALICE K. DORMANN

Extraverts communicate one-on-one or in groups with equal ease. They enjoy talking and bouncing their ideas off of others. Airing a thought that isn't fully formed doesn't faze an Extravert, who develops ideas and gains clarity through verbalizing. Mulling things over privately (the Introvert's preferred strategy) doesn't work well for the Extravert. Although it may be difficult for others to get a word in edgewise, Extraverts genuinely welcome input from many different sources. Usually, however, they aren't really seeking advice: hearing their thoughts out loud helps them find clarity.

> How can I tell what I think till I see what I say?
>
> E. M. FORSTER

In their eagerness to interact, Extraverts often don't carefully consider what they're saying before the words come tumbling out of their mouths. Contrary to appearances, however, they're not completely lacking in internal judgment about what is or is not appropriate to say. But because they have a hard time restraining themselves, Extraverts tend to make impromptu comments that have unintended consequences or implications.

Extraverts think fast and talk faster. Enthusiastic and expressive conversationalists, they grow even more energized as the discussion develops. Some Extraverts forget that communication is a back-and-forth proposition: often talking more than they listen, they can dominate conversations.

> If other people are going to talk,
> conversation becomes impossible.
>
> JAMES MCNEIL WHISTLER

Extraverts grow uncomfortable with long gaps in a conversation. To end the silence, they'll fill in the space with the first thing that comes

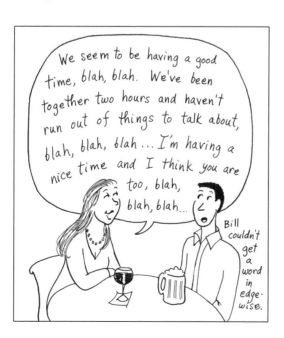

to mind; even an inappropriate remark or inane babble is fine with them—at least it's not silence! Paired with a more introverted companion, the Extravert tends to take over the conversation, talking on instead of waiting patiently for the other person to participate.

Extraverts often like being around other Extraverts; the quick exchanges of words galvanize their energy. When one Extravert wants to say something to another Extravert, he or she just chimes in without hesitation: neither party worries about interrupting the other's flow of thought or about their remarks being misperceived. In fact, Extraverts are sometimes overtly competitive with each other for airtime.

> If you think before you speak, the
> other fellow gets in his joke first.
>
> ED HOWE

Of course, not all Extraverts are obsessive talkers. To get the idea across, I'm describing the extreme end of the extraversion spectrum. Keep in mind that this preference is expressed somewhere along a continuum from mild to extreme.

Extraverts at Work

Extraverts thrive in an active, stimulating environment where they have the opportunity to interact with many people. Working as part of a team or in a busy office suits most Extraverts best. Extraverts would suffer from boredom, tedium, and low energy if stuck in a room working alone all day. Most jobs do have some introverted activities—writing reports, filing papers, making calculations, and so on. An Extravert is usually better off performing such tasks around other people, if the work doesn't require deep concentration.

With their strong verbal skills and outward show of confidence, Extraverts do well at marketing and promoting themselves. They

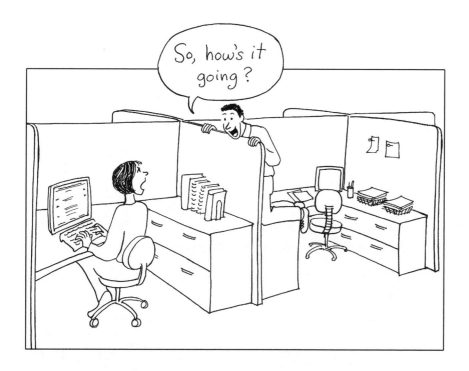

prefer to be in the limelight and aren't as drawn to working behind the scenes.

Famous Extraverts

Dr. Phil, Katie Couric, Larry King, Steve Martin, Bill Clinton,
Joe Biden, Sarah Palin, Whoopi Goldberg, Joan Rivers,
Dave Letterman, Newt Gingrich, John F. Kennedy,
Jim Carey, Dolly Parton, Tony Robbins, Donald Trump,
Robin Williams, Jack Nicholson, Arsenio Hall

I like to do all the talking myself. It saves
time and prevents arguments.

MARGARET THATCHER

What Drives an Extravert Crazy

- Waiting forever for someone to answer a question, because he or she has to think of the perfect way to respond

- People who are stingy with their conversation, as though it were made of gold

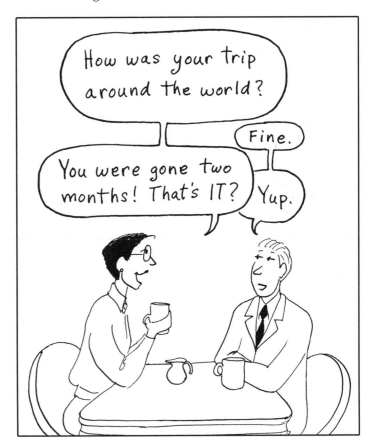

- Work that is slow-paced or offers little opportunity for interaction with others

- Antisocial people who don't understand the value of good company—or bad company, for that matter (in a pinch, an Extravert will chat up a telemarketer)

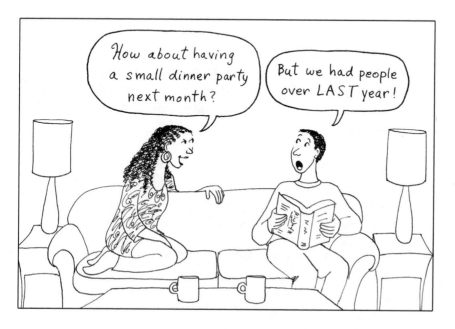

- People who are always trying to protect their "space"

- People who rarely take the initiative to reach out

- The silent treatment

I'm an Extravert. Now What?

Now that you know what type you are, these tips will help you own your type, recognize your limitations, and improve all your interactions with the world.

- Practice thinking before speaking. It's wonderful to be articulate, but having a direct line from your thoughts to your mouth isn't always a good idea.

> Often the difference between a successful
> marriage and a mediocre one consists of leaving
> about three or four things a day unsaid.
>
> HARLAN MILLER

- As you speak, take notice of your listener's interest level. If the person isn't talking or responding, pause and allow time for silence. If you see yawns and hear snoring, it may be time to stop.

- Avoid dominating conversations or turning them into monologues. For example, when a friend or co-worker asks how your weekend was, share an interesting tidbit—and then ask about theirs. (And remember to listen to the answer.)

- Keep in mind that your ideas are interesting, but so are those of other people.

> In conversation keep in mind that
> you're more interested in what you
> have to say than anyone else.
>
> ANDY ROONEY

- Every now and then, direct your attention to the volume of your voice. If the decibel level is rattling the walls, speak a little more softly.

- Avoid overcommitting yourself. Too many activities and events can leave you feeling scattered or stressed. Try to focus on what is most meaningful to you.

- Be careful of becoming so busy that you neglect those who are important to you.

- Try occasionally engaging in activities that do not involve being with others—reading, crafts, gardening, meditating, and so on.

What a lovely surprise to discover how
un-lonely being alone can be.

ELLEN BURSTYN

- When you're feeling low, seek out the company of other Extraverts to recharge your batteries.

You Might Be an Introvert If . . .

- Your three favorite companions are named me, myself, and I.

- You have found yourself hiding in the bathroom at a party more than once.

- A good vacation is being at home with your books and videos.

- When you call someone, you hope you get their answering machine.

- You break into a puddle of sweat when your turn to share in a circle is approaching.

- You cringe when someone takes the stationary bike next to yours at the gym.

- Your closest friend hasn't heard from you in months.

- Carpooling, even with someone you like, is never your preference.

- In your office there's a physical barrier (such as a large desk or table) between you and a client.

A barber asked King Archelaus
how he would like his hair cut.
"In silence," replied the king.

ARCHELAUS, RULED 413–399 BC

Introverts at Their Best	Introverts at Their Worst
Quiet	Distant
Calm demeanor	Detached
Independent	Unsociable
Self-sufficient	Aloof
Content being on their own	Withdrawn
Slow-paced	Guarded
Think before speaking	Passive
A bit mysterious	Too quiet

Introverts 101

Introverts focus their attention on their inner world of ideas, impressions, feelings, and thoughts. They need plenty of time on their own to reflect upon and internalize information. This is what energizes them. If they don't get enough alone time, they feel depleted and drained. Introverts simply don't need as much external stimulation as Extraverts do. It's not that they don't enjoy being with others, but companionship is satisfying to them only for limited periods. After spending time with another person, no matter how gratifying the experience, they need to recharge. It's as if the energy they have spent interacting with another person now needs to be replenished in solitude.

> I love people. I love my family, my children
> . . . but inside myself is a place where I
> live all alone and that's where you renew
> your springs that never dry up.
>
> PEARL S. BUCK

Too much stimulation from the outside world can feel overwhelming for an Introvert. To protect their inner world from what is sometimes perceived as an invasion, they tend to maintain a certain distance and separation.

Introverts often enjoy solo activities—reading, being on the computer, watching TV, going to a movie alone, or even traveling alone. They may also prefer individual sports like running, swimming, or taking long hikes in nature. For a few Introverts, the preference for solitude extends to living alone.

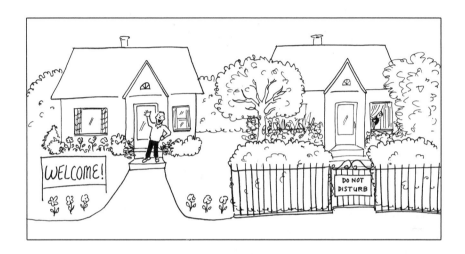

Social Life

The reluctance of Introverts to initiate contact with others doesn't mean they don't care. Sometimes they find it just too awkward or uncomfortable to reach out, even to those they feel deeply about. For many Introverts it can understandably take a great deal of emotional energy to just pick up the phone and make a call.

The discomfort of Introverts around strangers, or even acquaintances, can be hard for Extraverts to understand. Just going out for dinner with someone they don't know that well creates anxiety beforehand and exhaustion afterward. Their reluctant and hesitant interactions with others can make them appear distant or unfriendly.

Introverts are not usually drawn to big social events, and they cannot comprehend why others are. At a wedding, dinner party, or any other gathering of more than two or three people, an Introvert can feel more like a spectator than a participant. Small talk and brief, superficial conversations not only make Introverts quite uncomfortable but bore and tire them as well. In large groups of people who share a great deal of extraverted energy, it is especially difficult for Introverts to connect. Occasionally, an Introvert will make a huge effort to match the energy in the room, but the strategy seldom works, and he or she winds up feeling even more empty and disconnected.

> I know the dying process begins the minute we are born, but sometimes it accelerates during dinner parties.
>
> CAROL MATTHAU

Meeting potential partners in the setting of a singles event can be challenging, to say the least, and it can be especially tortuous for an Introvert. Anxiety runs especially high for male Introverts, since men are traditionally expected to initiate contact—not an Introvert's strongest ability. Some brave souls will take the risk of introducing themselves to others, but such overtures do not come naturally. Because it's so difficult to work up a head of steam and charge forward, unattached Introverts tend to date less than their unattached extraverted counterparts. Online dating has made it easier for Introverts to connect—but eventually they have to meet face-to-face.

Don't be surprised, however, if you see an Introvert completely relaxed and at ease in an intimate conversation with those he or she knows well. In fact, it is not uncommon to observe an Introvert happily engaged with one or two close companions, maybe in an out-of-the-way corner or out on a back porch. In such situations, the Introvert may even look like a social butterfly, but it may take this person a long time afterward to recharge his or her "social reserves."

Introverts often feel more relaxed and at ease at social events when they have a clear-cut role to play, such as registering people for a class, serving as an officer of an organization, or helping with the food preparation at a party.

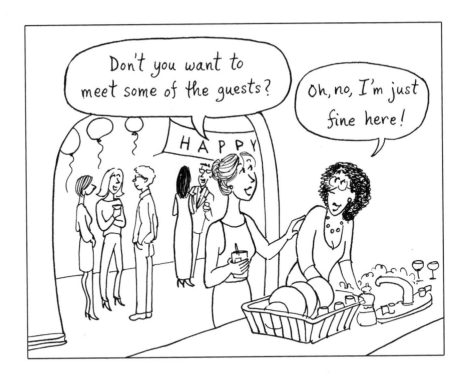

Introverts also feel more comfortable with others when they're engaging in pastimes that don't require a great deal of conversation, like hiking, playing tennis, or seeing a movie. Activities like these provide a structure for interacting with others. It eases the Introvert into feeling connected without as much pressure to talk or interact. The Introvert can just *be*.

Even though Introverts can entertain themselves easily enough, they usually enjoy having a close friend or partner as a companion for some of their activities. One-on-one connecting comes most naturally for them. They usually prefer this type of relating over relating to groups or parties. They also tend to feel more comfortable in a group if they are with someone instead of alone. Having a companion not only provides them with a buffer but gives them the sense that they belong. Sometimes being with just one other person is energizing and comforting for an Introvert.

For an Introvert who craves company but still needs to retain some sense of boundaries, being with another Introvert is the perfect solution. That human being is present, but not intruding on their space.

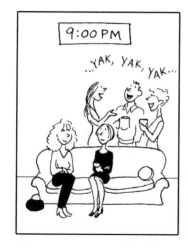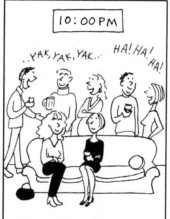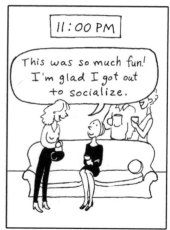

Being with an Extravert appeals to some Introverts because they can just listen and don't have to talk. The Extravert fills in gaps in conversations and also is more likely to initiate social contact. But the downside of such a relationship is that a strong Extravert can provide a running commentary on . . . everything.

Communicating with an Introvert

Introverts tend to be reserved, private, and self-contained. They often prefer to just stand back and observe, especially in new or unfamiliar situations. You might interpret their silence as boredom or lack of interest, but that's not always the case. Introverts just don't feel a strong need to externalize their thoughts or feelings. They'll answer your questions politely enough, but won't go into much depth unless they know you well. They are certainly capable of opening up to others, but they usually feel close to only a select few. In fact, some Introverts have only one or two good friends—a situation with which they are perfectly content. Having a large social circle is the last thing an Introvert wants. It's just too time-consuming and draining to keep up that many relationships.

Introverts can feel overwhelmed by other people's ideas and energy. Rather than discussing or hashing out an issue, they might prefer to take in information and then process it alone. Once they've had time to think the matter through, they're more willing to share their thoughts and opinions. And the more time they have to deliberate, the more confident they feel about sharing their ideas and opinions.

> Time spent in silent deliberation is better than time spent with one's foot in one's mouth.
>
> LUNA BARON

Contrary to appearances, however, Introverts have as many ideas, emotions, and opinions as Extraverts; it just all goes on inside of them. And even though they don't say that much, they can be very involved in a conversation as they make all kinds of associations, comparing and contrasting the situations, people, and experiences under discussion with other situations, people, and experiences they have known.

When Introverts perceive that someone is interested in what they have to say, or when they feel knowledgeable about the subject, they can be quite talkative. Still, because they don't share themselves so readily, Introverts—especially those with a strong tendency toward introversion—can be difficult to get to know.

All of us occasionally play the game of "what I should have said," but no one plays it as well, or as frequently, as the Introvert, whose best conversations often occur after the fact, when he or she is alone again. Needless to say, Introverts often wish they could get their ideas out more forcefully, and in a timelier way.

Introverts at Work

Most Introverts prefer working independently in a quiet environment that is conducive to concentration. They don't mind associating with others when they need support, but as soon as they feel confident about what they're doing, they're ready to move off and work independently. Collaborating is fine on occasion, but they're usually more interested in connecting with the task than with their colleagues.

If they like their job, Introverts work happily for long periods of time without communication or encouragement from others. Unlike Extraverts, they need little or no feedback about their work—unless they're feeling insecure. Because of their ability to focus deeply, Introverts sometimes become so immersed in an activity that they are oblivious to what is happening around them.

In general, Introverts are less likely than Extraverts to volunteer for or take a leadership role. In most situations, they're much happier staying in the background, working behind the scenes, and not bringing attention to themselves. Introverts can, however, be strong and inspiring leaders—Al Gore, Gandhi, and President Barack Obama come to mind. Introverts make up a slight majority of the upper levels of government, the military, and the corporate world, despite being only 25 to 30 percent of the population.

Famous Introverts

John McCain, Thomas Jefferson, Abraham Lincoln, Martin Luther King Jr., Meryl Streep, James Bond, Tiger Woods, Johnny Carson, Jerry Seinfeld, Steven Spielberg, James Dean, Jackie Kennedy

> If you are lonely while you're alone,
> you are in bad company.
>
> JEAN-PAUL SARTRE

What Drives an Introvert Crazy

- Chatterboxes who dominate the conversation

> I haven't spoken to my wife in years—
> I didn't want to interrupt her.
>
> RODNEY DANGERFIELD

- Being made the center of attention without warning (or even *with* warning, for that matter!)

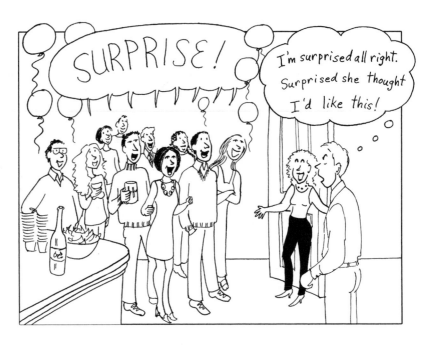

- People who are oblivious to all the subtle—and not so subtle—signs that others don't want to interact

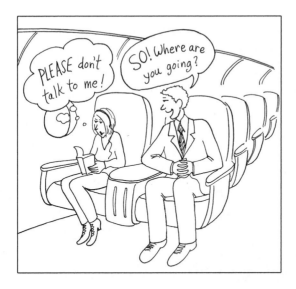

- Multitasking junkies who can't give full attention to any one thing—or person

- Having to listen to someone ramble on endlessly

- Being pressured to talk

- Getting nonverbal signals when you don't talk or respond quickly that you may be dull or stupid

- Discovering that others are discussing their personal life

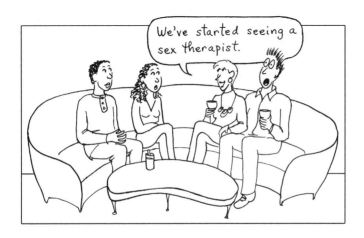

I'm an Introvert. Now What?

- Create a retreat that's all yours—perhaps your bedroom, but even a broom closet will do. No one is allowed in unless you invite them. For you, time alone is not a luxury—it's a necessity in order for you to feel comfortable in the world.

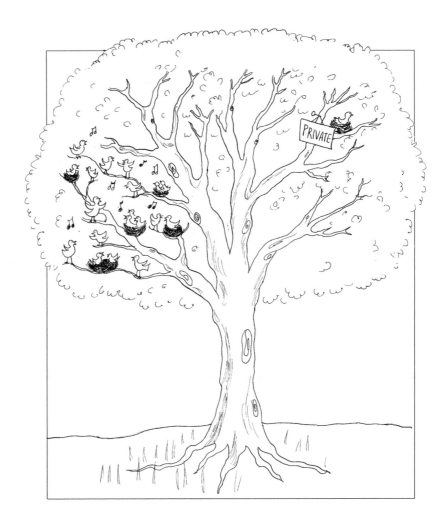

- If you work with others, find ways to take off by yourself during the day—maybe going for a walk during your lunch hour or break time—so that you can recharge.

- Remember that you are not the only one who might feel awkward in social situations. Sometimes just being honest about how you are feeling is the best icebreaker.

- Take the initiative in reaching out to people instead of waiting for others to ask you to join them. Once in a while, push yourself to take more social risks.

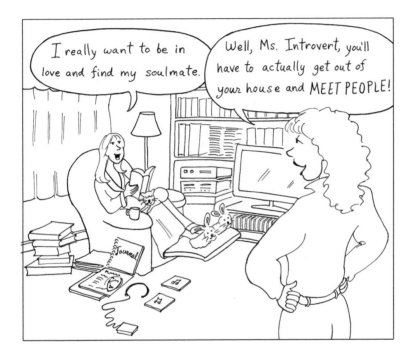

- Be more generous with compliments and praise. When people are important to you, let them know.

Silent gratitude isn't much use to anyone.

ANONYMOUS

- If you're having a disagreement and find yourself at a loss for words, don't abandon the issue. Instead, try saying something like: "I need some time to myself so I can get more clear."

- Keep in mind that your inner dialogue may be so real to you that you think you've verbalized your ideas to others. In actuality, you may have shared only a tiny part of what you think you said.

- Try doing some of your thinking out loud. Verbalize rough drafts of thoughts that you end up changing.

- In group conversations, volunteer your ideas so that people don't miss out on your usually well-thought-out contributions. Even though a point may seem obvious to you, it's often not so to others.

- Initiate discussions rather than always waiting for others to drag things out of you.

- Recognize and appreciate the difference between healthy solitude and unnecessary isolation.

Language has created the word
"loneliness" to express the pain of
being alone, and the word "solitude" to
express the glory of being alone.

PAUL TILLICH

4

The Extravert/Introvert Relationship

The saying "opposites attract" is never truer than when an Extravert and Introvert fall in love. The Extravert often finds the Introvert's calm, cool demeanor and somewhat mysterious quality appealing, and the Introvert's ability and willingness to listen is especially attractive. The Introvert often finds the Extravert entertaining and charming. The Introvert particularly admires the Extravert's ease in relating to and conversing with others, in distinct contrast to the Introvert's more reserved style.

In the beginning, both are more likely to enjoy being "just the two of us" than they will be later in the relationship. At this time, the Extravert may try to be a more attentive listener, making sure not to interrupt or to pressure the Introvert to converse. The Introvert, on the other hand, is likely to start the relationship by making an effort to be more social, even going so far as to initiate plans. In time, however, the couple's natural preferences will reassert themselves. The Extravert will want to interact with more people, while the Introvert will want more time alone. Eventually, the Extravert's need for interaction versus the Introvert's need for solitude may cause them to move in opposite directions. Attempts to coerce an Introvert partner into behaving more like an Extravert almost always backfire, as do any efforts on the part of the Introvert to place a damper on the Extravert's more outgoing and energetic style.

This dysfunctional dynamic is especially strong when each partner has a relatively extreme preference on the Extravert-Introvert scale. Many couples with more moderate preferences find it easier to compromise around their differing needs for interaction and privacy. But even those with strong opposing preferences are capable of moving closer to the center of the continuum on occasion and may find that their relationship improves when they do. It's important that each partner keep in mind that extraversion and introversion are natural preferences, not deliberate strategies to drive each other crazy.

Couples with the same preference on this dimension have an advantage over those who do not. Partners who share a preference for either extraversion or introversion will have a much easier time in some ways. (The alignment of their other three preferences will also have an effect on their overall compatibility.) Two Extraverts tend to be socially active and energetic and are likely to enjoy a busy lifestyle. Verbally they're a good match, both being talkative, fond of lively discussions, eager to bounce their ideas off of each other, and accustomed to thinking out loud. Both share an enthusiastic approach to most activities in life. They have similar needs for social interaction and being with many different people, but one member of the pair—the stronger Extravert—will most likely want more activity and interaction than the other.

On the downside, two Extraverts who are romantically involved can become so overextended with activities and social obligations that they forget to spend time together.

Two Introverts can also get along well. Each respects the other's need for quiet and privacy. Neither has an urgent need to socialize, but both will occasionally enjoy being with a small group of low-key friends. They understand each other's desire to spend time alone, and neither of them will pressure the other to entertain or be with other people. Two Introverts usually enjoy reading and relaxing and spending time at home. Quiet, often nonverbal companionship can be very satisfying to Introverts, who do not consider silence boring and see nothing wrong with not wanting to be with others.

On the downside, in a relationship in which neither partner initiates social activities, too much isolation (even for an Introvert) may be the result. The Introvert couple avoids becoming too insular when one partner—the one with the more moderate preference—gravitates (consciously or otherwise) toward a more extraverted role and maintains contact with friends and family.

Critical to meeting the challenges of the opposite-preference relationship is an understanding that the preferences are natural to who we are. What often occurs when we are less judgmental about ways of being that differ from our own is greater acceptance and understanding. In fact, an Extravert/Introvert relationship has much to offer those who are open to personal growth. Each partner can count on the other's strengths to compensate for and supplement their own weaknesses. And it is more than possible for each to learn to embody the positive opposite qualities they see in the other.

Still, the Extravert/Introvert couple will face challenges. Like any other relationship issue, having a different preference than your partner may make you want to tear out your hair (or theirs). But if you're willing to invest some effort in bridging the gap between the two of you, the payoff can make your work well worthwhile. Extraverts and Introverts can certainly find harmonious ways to live and love together. Sometimes it is important for one partner to give in and go with the other's desires; when this happens, the favor is likely to be returned. Instead of growing apart, the Extravert/Introvert couple can find interests that they share, such as walking the dog, reading the newspaper together, sharing or watching TV shows, hiking, or taking a meditation class.

I have found the following techniques to be effective in improving communication, decreasing stress, and increasing respect between Extravert/Introvert partners.

How to Get Along with an Extravert

- Appreciate the enthusiasm, energy, and bursts of outright excitement that an Extravert brings to the relationship.

- It's difficult (maybe even impossible) to praise an Extravert too much. Compliment your Extravert partner often—as well as out loud and in front of other people—on his or her appearance, accomplishments, and achievements. (Also say nice things behind the Extravert's back. Word is sure to get back to your partner . . . almost as quickly as it does when you criticize him or her).

- Understand that an Extravert's desire to share personal news—good or bad—with lots of people doesn't mean that he or she doesn't love or rely on you immensely. It's just the Extravert's nature to spread any story far and wide.

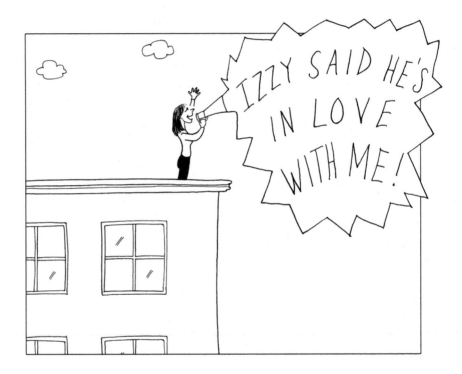

- Keep in mind that an Extravert figures things out by talking. The thoughts he or she verbalizes are often more like a first draft than a final report. Don't expect pearls of wisdom right off the bat.

- Accompany your Extravert partner to social events and activities every now and then. You don't have to keep up with your partner's whirlwind schedule, but it's a nice gesture to go along once in a while. As you know, Extraverts take great pleasure in companionship, and your partner will appreciate the effort. And who knows—you might have more fun than you imagined.

- Don't pressure your Extravert partner to leave a party or other event before he or she is ready. Some Extravert/Introvert couples drive separately to events just so that both can exit at whatever time they please.

- Understand the Extravert's need to spend time with people other than you. Ideally, you'll even encourage your partner to do this. This need is simply a reflection of the Extravert's inner wiring, not a statement about your relationship. Just as plants need water, your Extravert needs frequent contact with loved ones.

- It's important to give Extraverts the time they require to express themselves. They have a lot to say, and they seldom say it concisely. So when your long-winded lover launches into yet another story, take a deep breath, relax, and remind yourself that you have a few quirks too.

- If all the verbiage gets to be too much for you, let your partner know . . . in a diplomatic way, of course. "I love you, honey, but I need to be quiet right now" conveys your point—and your affection. "You talk too much"—not so much.

- Verbalize what you're feeling as you're feeling it some of the time, especially when you're being physically intimate. Don't assume that your feelings of pleasure or love are being communicated some other way. Your Extravert partner may interpret your silence as boredom or disinterest, even when this is not the case.

- Don't give your partner the dreaded silent treatment when you're upset or angry. Share your thoughts and reactions and be forthcoming about what's going on with you. This can be a real stretch for an Introvert, but in the long run it's one of the most helpful things you can do for your relationship.

- When conflicts arise, agree on a time to talk over the issues and make sure you follow through. That way, you get the time you need to think things through, while your partner is reassured that you're not simply withdrawing.

Statements That Extraverts Hate to Hear

"Do you always have to be doing something?"
"Could you tone it down a bit?"
"Zip your lip!"
"Calm down."
"You never shut up!"

How to Get Along with an Introvert

- Don't drag a reluctant Introvert to social engagements or make him feel guilty for not accompanying you. Instead, make it easy for your partner to opt out if he's tired or not interested. Sample script: "I'd love to have your company, honey, but I completely understand if you'd rather not go." Follow up with a kiss or a reassuring hug. Then, when you reconnect, a cloud of resentment won't be hanging overhead.

Some people ask the secret of our long marriage.
We take time to go to a restaurant two times
a week. A little candlelight, dinner, soft music,
and dancing. She goes Tuesdays, I go Fridays.

HENNY YOUNGMAN

- Respect the Introvert's need for privacy and solitude and don't take it personally. Unlike you, your introverted partner replenishes his or her energy most effectively by spending time alone. Don't panic—your partner will emerge from the cocoon of solitude refreshed and ready to engage again.

- Don't depend on an Introvert to meet all of your companionship needs.

- When you invite an Introvert to a party or other social event, provide that person with advance information. Introverts feel more comfortable about saying yes if they know how long the occasion will last, who will be there, and other reassuring details.

- At an event, be sure to introduce Introverts to people they are likely to enjoy talking to and help them ease into the conversation. (Sample script: "Mary, I'd like you to meet Martha; she's a big fan of flamenco dancing, just like you.")

- If you have planned a "just the two of us" activity, avoid turning it into a "just the three of us" (or "just the twenty of us") occasion.

- Pass on social activities sometimes and make a little more room for the relationship.

- Cultivate a higher level of comfort with quiet. Spend some of your couple time in silence—reading, listening to music, or doing other things "together alone." Your Introvert partner can feel a close connection even when neither of you say a word.

Silences make the real conversations between friends.

MARGARET LEE RUNBECK

- Don't spoil an intimate moment with chatter. What you think of as communication or self-expression may be perceived by your partner as redundant, superficial, or meaningless babble.

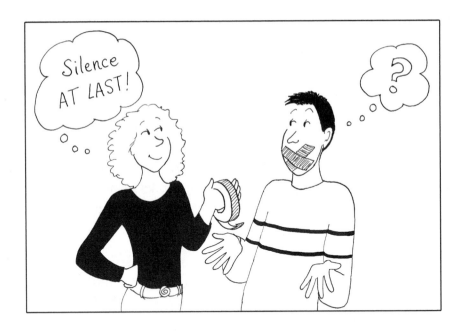

- Try not to repeat yourself. You don't have to take a vow of silence, but when you can manage it, your partner will appreciate a more minimalist conversational style.

Married couples who love each other tell each
other a thousand things without talking.

CHINESE PROVERB

- Step one: draw out an Introvert by asking thoughtful, nonintrusive questions. Step two: really listen to the answers. Everyone, especially Introverts, will appreciate this kind of focused attention, but beyond that, many Introverts have an aversion to repeating themselves. If you pay close attention, they won't have to.

- Be patient with a slow-paced conversational style and frequent pauses. If you're a typical Extravert, you probably take up a lot of clock time too—your verbal style just includes more words.

> The opposite of talking isn't listening.
> The opposite of talking is waiting.
>
> FRAN LEBOWITZ

- When important issues arise, give your Introvert partner plenty of time to ponder before sitting down to talk. Although you may feel impatient, it's counterproductive to press for an immediate response. Your partner will be more forthcoming if he or she has time to consider the situation carefully.

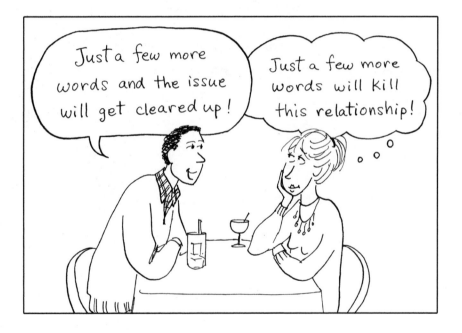

- Don't assume that the silence of an Introvert signals stubbornness, willfulness, or lack of interest.

- Respect the Introvert's need for privacy—both spatial and psychological. It may not seem like a big deal to you to tell a friend about your partner's family history or to discuss his or her weight problem. To the Introvert, however, this type of discussion with a third party can feel like a major betrayal.

- Don't praise Introverts too much in public or call attention to them in other ways. The spotlight is not a comfortable place for them.

Statements That Introverts Hate to Hear

"Come out of your shell."

"Don't be shy."

"Why are you so quiet?"

"What's on your mind?"

"What's wrong?"

"Why won't you come join us?"

"Why can't you just smile?"

"Cat got your tongue?"

"Do you *ever* talk?"

5

The Perceiving Preference

SENSORS/INTUITIVES

Read the following statements and check the sentence that describes you best—A or B. To achieve the most accurate score, answer the statements according to what is true for you, not according to what you would like to be true or think ought to be true.

The Inventory

1. A ☐ I tend to be more realistic, practical, and down-to-earth than imaginative.

   B ☒ I tend to be more imaginative, innovative, and creative than realistic.

2. A ☐ I prefer information that is concrete and factual.

   B ☒ I prefer information that is abstract and theoretical.

3. A ☐ Rather than speculating about the future, I like to focus on what is at hand in the present.

   B ☒ I enjoy thinking about new possibilities and ideas; my attention is drawn to what might be or could be in the future.

4. A ☐ I pay more attention to details and specifics than to the big picture.

   B ☒ I pay more attention to the big picture than to details and specifics.

5. A ☐ I don't have a strong need to change or improve what already exists. I'm usually content to just let things be.

   B ☒ I tend to look for ways to improve upon things and enjoy doing them in new ways.

6. A ☐ I know what's going on just by observing and using my common sense.

   B ☒ My intuition tells me much of what I need to know.

7. A ☐ My favorite tasks are practical and produce tangible results.

   B ☒ My favorite tasks involve imagination and innovation.

8. A ☐ I tend to interpret other people's statements and actions at face value rather than trying to "read between the lines."

   B ☒ I tend to look for the underlying meaning of what other people say or do.

9. A ☐ I am bothered by people who always want to improve things and do them in new ways.

   B ☒ I am bothered by people who give blow-by-blow descriptions of the details.

10. A ☐ I am more interested in facts than theories.

    B ☒ I am more interested in theories than facts.

Scoring

In the first blank space below, record how many times you chose A as the answer to one of these ten questions. In the second blank space below, record how many times you chose B.

Total

___0___ A Sensor

___10___ B Intuitive

Sensors and Intuitives in a Nutshell

The third set of preferences refers to how we take in information and perceive the world. Sensors obtain information mainly through the five senses—what they see, hear, taste, touch, and smell in the "real" world. They focus on what is concrete and tangible, what actually exists, here and now. Intuitives also take in information through the five senses, just as all human beings do, but they pay more attention to hunches and insights—the sixth sense, so to speak. They are most at home in the realm of ideas and imagination.

Your preference on the sensing-intuiting dimension not only is linked to your perception of reality but also affects your style of communication, your career choices, and many other important aspects of life. Yet because sensing and intuition manifest themselves internally, they are sometimes difficult to discern. There are not many outer cues that can help us determine preferences—whether our own or someone else's—on this dimension.

As with the other sets of preferences, we all have aspects of both sensing and intuiting within ourselves. What differs from person to person is the degree to which we rely on sensing or intuiting and, correspondingly, our level of comfort with each preference and how effectively they work for us. We need a balance within ourselves of both sensing (to keep ourselves grounded in reality) and intuiting (to help us look to future possibilities).

Because the percentage of Sensors in the U.S. population is so much higher than the percentage of Intuitives (65 to 75 percent are Sensors, while 25 to 35 percent are Intuitives), our culture generally gives greater value to the perceptions of Sensors. If you happen to be in the minority on this one, you're probably already aware of that fact on some level. But once again, it's not better to be a Sensor than an Intuitive, nor is it better to be an Intuitive than a Sensor. Both preferences are associated with some wonderful qualities, and both are associated with certain liabilities.

Because Sensors and Intuitives see the world in fundamentally different ways, communication between them can be difficult and awkward. Miscommunications abound, sometimes so much so that it seems as though they are speaking different languages. Since the two perceptions of reality are so different, a strong Sensor and a strong Intuitive rarely see eye to eye. Both firmly believe that their perceptions are more accurate and valid than the other's and that their innate skills are superior. Differences in this set of preferences can be a source of frustration, irritation, and conflict, especially between those people who have pronounced leanings toward one side or the other.

SENSORS

You Might Be a Sensor If . . .

- You relish living your life, not just dreaming about what you'll do in the future.

- "Tried and true" is one of your favorite mottos. "If it ain't broke, don't fix it" is another.

- All that talk about the meaning of life—what does it really *mean*?

- Doing something that always works the same way you've always done it puts a big smile on your face.

- When you stop to smell the roses, you actually *smell* the roses.

- When your boss says, "Let's brainstorm a little," you say to yourself, *Oh, no, let's not.*

- You think sex is sex, and philosophy is philosophy.

- Your holiday decorations haven't changed since 1982.

- When you find an article that refutes a friend's crazy new theory, you can't wait to bring it to his or her attention.

- "Good common sense" is your middle name.

Sensors at Their Best	Sensors at Their Worst
Practical	Uninspired
Pragmatic	Nearsighted
Down to earth	Unimaginative
Realistic	Overly detail-oriented
Sensible	Lacking vision
Grounded	Conventional
Fully present in the here and now	Can't see the forest for the trees
Attentive to the immediate needs of self and others	Fearful of change

Sensors 101

We live in a fantasy world, a world of illusion.
The great task in life is to find reality.

IRIS MURDOCH

Sensors, just as the term implies, are all about their senses. As far as most are concerned, there's no such thing as a *sixth* sense, but they're deeply tuned in to the basic five. In fact, Sensors take in information mainly through these physical sources of perception by what they can see, hear, taste, touch, and smell. Of course, you don't have to be a Sensor to rely on your senses, as we all do myriad times every day. Testing the temperature of the bathwater, listening to the rain on the roof, savoring that first sip of morning coffee, making love with your partner . . . in all of these activities, we perceive the world through our physical senses. Sensors, however, focus intently on such sense-based experiences.

Here and now is what matters to the Sensor, not what will happen next. Rather than anticipating what *might* be or *could* be, they focus on what *is*. Sensors are often keen observers of their physical surroundings.

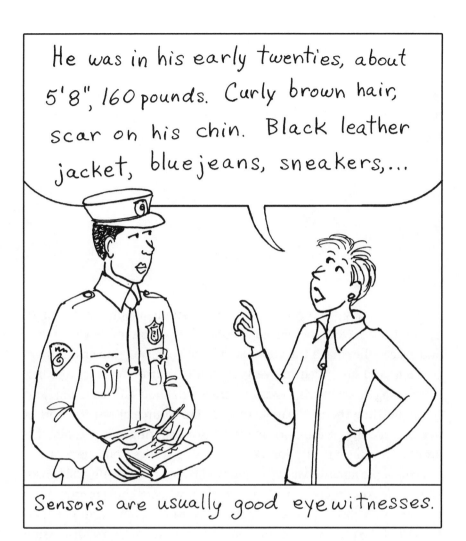

Although not much given to introspection, daydreaming, or musing about the mysteries of existence, Sensors do not lack an intuitive side. But for them, intuition and imagination take a back seat to observation.

Although Sensors are good at managing the real world with relative ease and skill, they can pay a penalty for ignoring their inner promptings, which, when ignored, can gradually fade away. When they do get an insight or a hunch, they often dismiss what might be important information. Their hunches and insights can be quite accurate, however, once they have a solid base in facts.

Communicating with a Sensor

Sensors express themselves clearly, in specific and uncomplicated terms; they prefer that others do the same. Sensors have sequential thoughts—one thought follows the next.

He liked to go from A to B without inventing letters in between.

JOHN MCPHEE

Sensors enjoy participating in conversations about the details of events they have experienced, people they know or have known, and places they have traveled to. Favored topics of conversation are concrete and grounded in everyday reality: current events, weather, prices, wages, accidents, disasters, trends in food and clothing, and so on. Reading the newspaper, an abundant source of just this sort of detail, is a daily pleasure for many Sensors; sharing snippets aloud is another. Sensors are also fond of recounting stories from the past.

If the topic remains vague or removed from ordinary life, the Sensor is likely to lose interest. And on occasion, when a conversation veers too far in an abstract direction, the Sensor may even misunderstand the gist of the communication. Some Sensors are capable of discussing abstract ideas, but this is not the most comfortable realm for them, and they'll do their best to shift such conversations in a more concrete and "sensible" direction.

Sensors' sentences are often direct and to the point. They tend to use conventional vocabulary and phrasing. Using metaphor or analogy and engaging in flights of fancy are just not the style of these feet-on-the-ground folks—but being extremely literal is. Sensors are also fond of comparisons, usually offered in a tone of complete self-assurance: "Stick shift is better than automatic," or "Eighty cents a pound is okay, but ninety-eight is ridiculous." Some Sensors also reflexively sprinkle their speech with clichés, old sayings, and proverbs, such as:

What you don't know can't hurt you.

You can't teach an old dog new tricks.

There's no such thing as a free lunch.

Two wrongs don't make a right.

Sensors are capable of storing an enormous amount of information on topics that interest them, and they can readily and accurately recall it. Names, birthdays, sports statistics—into the Sensor's "data bank" go these facts, and out they come when needed.

Relating Intimately with a Sensor

Sensors view romantic relationships realistically, noting the positive and negative qualities of their partner (or potential partners) in the present moment. For Sensors, the rendezvous begins when the two people get together, not before. Daydreaming is more likely to occur *after* a first date, when there are real facts to draw on. Far from planning the honeymoon before the first date, the Sensor can't formulate a fantasy in the absence of concrete details.

The bad news about the Sensor as a romantic partner is that he or she is not likely to intuit your unspoken secret desires or sweep you off your feet with the most imaginative or creative gift you've ever received. The good news, on the other hand, is that this down-to-earth lover does not expect you to be a paragon of perfection. Nice and normal will do just fine, thank you. In a committed relationship, most Sensors are not inclined to wonder whether the grass is greener on the other side. When things go wrong in a relationship, Sensors are likely to face the facts directly. After all, they never expected perfection in the first place.

Some Sensors are traditionalists when it comes to settling down with a partner. No matter what the modern trend may be, most crave old-fashioned matrimony, complete with bridal showers, engagement and wedding rings, and, of course, a marriage certificate.

After the wedding, Sensors are not likely to read you love poems or spend time brainstorming about how to change the world or playing "a penny for your thoughts." You can count on the Sensor, however, to show in tangible ways that he or she cares—by mowing the lawn, repairing the roof, washing the car, cooking the meals, cleaning the house, or providing security and material comforts. And if an occasion calls for a card, a gift, flowers, a visit with extended family, or other traditional expressions of affection, most Sensors are happy to oblige.

Sensors often like doing what other people do and having what other people have. Many like talking about and taking care of their possessions.

Sensors at Work

Sensors like working in environments that produce practical or useful products or services. They are drawn to work that calls on attention to facts and details. Conversely, fields that involve abstract, theoretical, speculative, or conceptual thinking seldom appeal to the Sensor, unless the work helps to solve practical problems. Sensors learn about abstract or theoretical things by doing them.

The Sensor wants to learn a job skill and use it. He or she learns best through observation and firsthand experience. Unlike Intuitives, who enjoy dreaming up new ways of doing things, Sensors don't like to start from scratch. Instead, they enjoy using new applications for something that has already been invented or established, like running a franchise business rather than starting a new one.

Practice is the best of all instructors.

PUBLILIUS SYRUS

At work as at home, Sensors are deeply interested in continuity, and novelty for the sake of novelty does not appeal to them. Rather than adopting a new idea or technique, the Sensor will look at what has been tried in the past, analyze how it has worked and how it is working now, find out what others have done in similar circumstances, determine what problems have arisen, and so on. Only when there is concrete evidence that the proposed new way is superior to the old will the Sensor see the need to make a change. Even then, the Sensor may feel more comfortable continuing to do things "by the book." On the flip side, this conservative approach to change means that Sensors are unlikely to make frivolous changes even when pressed to do so.

Sensors are often thought of as the "can-do" guy or gal around the workplace. They are drawn to tasks or projects that can produce immediate and tangible results. Sensors are adept at quickly sizing up a situation and seeing what is inefficient and impractical, and they are realistic about resources, costs, and the time requirements of a project. In many work situations, a knack for collecting data and sorting out facts and figures makes the Sensor a valued player in the problem-solving process. Sensors often do well in crisis situations.

Famous Sensors

Liberace, Johnny Cash, Billy Graham, Lyndon Johnson, George Patton, Nancy Reagan, Paula Abdul, Kareem Abdul-Jabbar, Magic Johnson, Mike Wallace, Adam Sandler, Julia Child, Rachel Ray, George H. W. Bush, Sylvester Stallone

You can observe a lot just by watchin'.

YOGI BERRA

Just the facts, ma'am.

JOE FRIDAY

> All genuine knowledge originates
> in direct experience.
>
> MAO TSE-TUNG

What Drives a Sensor Crazy

- People who always want to improve upon things and do them in new ways

- People who overlook the details

- A lack of common sense

- People who speak in generalities rather than specifics

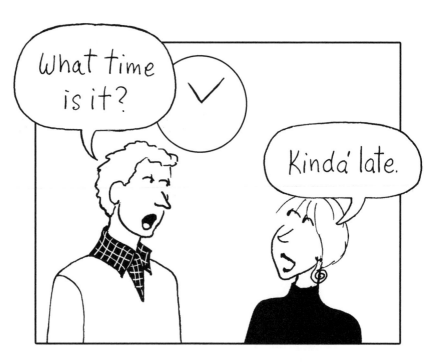

- Talking about doing something instead of doing it

- People who don't pay attention to what's right in front of them

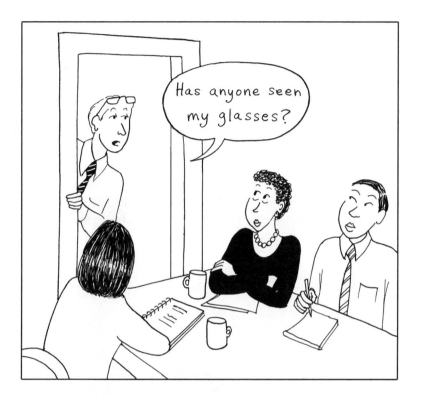

- Idealists, daydreamers, and everyone else who sees the world through rose-colored glasses

I'm a Sensor. Now What?

- Feed your senses. It's the best way to alleviate stress.

- To develop your Intuitive side, learn a little bit about ways of knowing that are unfamiliar to you—your hunches, intuitions, fantasies, and dreams.

- When problem-solving, be open to brainstorming with others. Try to consider ideas that seem impractical, even absurd. Remember times in the past when the unknown or unfamiliar led to a good outcome.

> Minds are like parachutes:
> they work best when open.
>
> LORD THOMAS DEWAR

- Nobody's better than you are at putting one foot in front of the other. For a change of pace (and altitude!), let your head float up in the clouds for a while.

- Avoid getting stuck in a rut and sticking with the same old routine *if* it's no longer working for you. Just because you've always done it one way doesn't mean that this is the only way to do it.

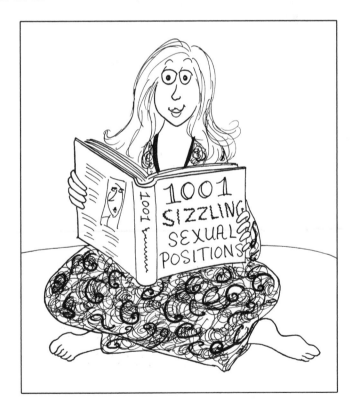

- When conflicts arise, the issues at hand often relate to a big-picture problem. Sensors squabble over small matters because they're uncomfortable (sometimes without even knowing it themselves) with more important matters. If you want to resolve a conflict, look at what's not being said—by you or by others.

- Make the most of your passion for the past by researching the history of your family. You'll enjoy the facts you uncover, and your work will be appreciated by generations to come.

- Go way out on a limb and sign up for a class in creative writing, philosophy, or music appreciation. Reading Carl Jung, Carlos Castaneda, or Gabriel Garcia Márquez is a good place to start. You may be surprised at what you discover.

- If spiritual exploration appeals to you, investigate one of the many Eastern philosophies that emphasize living in the here and now and focusing on the present moment.

You Might Be an Intuitive If . . .

- Vacationing at the beach, you're unaware of the gentle waves lapping at your feet as you stroll along the shore—you're too busy daydreaming about *next* year's vacation.

- You frequently find yourself thinking, *What if . . .?* and spinning an elaborate fantasy from there.

- It's hard for you to do something the same way twice.

- Your lover complains that you sometimes seem far away during intimate moments, as though you're thinking about something else.

- You could fall in love with someone you've never seen if they were to write you amazing letters.

- Given a choice between Einstein and Michelangelo's *David* as a life partner, you'd go for the genius, not the muscle man.

- Games of imagination (quick, fill in the blanks: "If I were a _Person_, I would _E taked or_") are usually easy for you—and of that Person. enjoyable.

- Okay, you admit it: every once in a while, you'd enjoy taking a vacation from your own hyperactive mind. But how exactly is that done?

Intuitives at Their Best	Intuitives at Their Worst
Imaginative ✓	Overly complex ✓
Innovative ✓	Impractical
Insightful ✓	Unrealistic ✓
Ingenious ✓	Unobservant
Original ✓	Overly idealistic ✓
Inquisitive ✓	Nonconcrete
Inventive ✓	Too speculative
Creative ✓	Starry-eyed
	Inattentive to details

Intuitives 101

> The world of reality has its limits;
> the world of imagination is boundless.
>
> JEAN-JACQUES ROUSSEAU

The Intuitive is like a TV satellite dish, tapping into many channels and signals beyond the local ones. Hunches, insights, and intuitive flashes—the Intuitive has access to all these sophisticated frequencies, yet is often oblivious to the basic information provided by the five senses. In distinct contrast to the experience of the Sensor (who is focused too much on concrete details), the big picture—what they call "the heart of the matter"—is everything to Intuitives. If they consider details at all, it is only after forming an idea of the big picture. As they take in information, Intuitives perceive patterns, relationships, and underlying meanings. A strong Intuitive, however, might not notice your new car or your new hairstyle. Intuitives are often bright, clever, fond of learning, and academically gifted. Many like knowledge for its own sake and enjoy continuous learning.

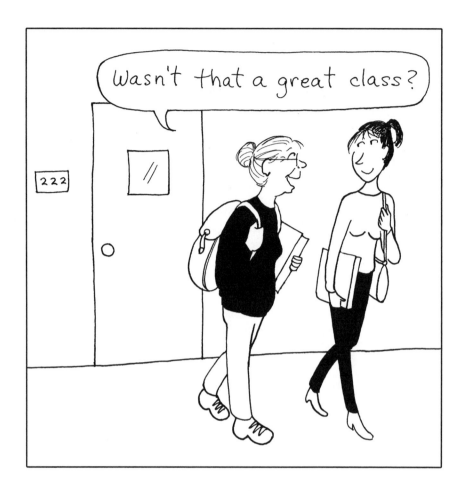

Intuitives are more strongly oriented toward what is possible than toward what is tangible. This does not mean that Intuitives lack a sensing side; it simply means that sensing takes a back seat to intuition. Being so focused on possibilities, the Intuitive sometimes discounts information that comes through direct observation and ends up with relatively undeveloped sensing abilities. In other words, imagination prevails at the expense of observation.

Intuitives face life expectantly—and face *is* the right word: they're excited about where they're going, not about where they've been. Much of their attention is focused on what *might* be or what *could* be, not on what *is*. Because they're so immersed in their thoughts and fantasies, they can come across as charmingly—or annoyingly—absentminded. When they attempt to remain grounded in the present, Intuitives are likely to become bored or frustrated. Some may be discontented with—or even acutely disturbed by—the constraints of day-to-day reality and will consequently speculate about *possible* (there's that word again!) ways to improve on it.

Reality can be beaten with enough imagination.

ANONYMOUS

Some Intuitives become so wrapped up in ideas and plans for the future that they neglect or ignore situations that require immediate attention in the present.

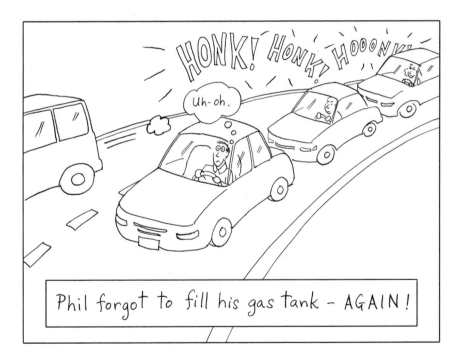

Phil forgot to fill his gas tank - AGAIN!

Communicating with an Intuitive

The Intuitive communicates in a more complicated, circuitous manner than the Sensor does. Thought and speech progress by leaps and bounds rather than in a linear step-by-step way. Typically, the Intuitive

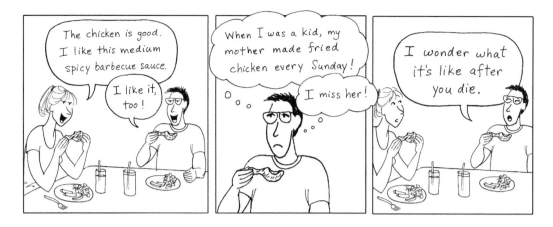

moves quickly from discussing the components and details of an issue to making generalizations, pointing out patterns, and finding hidden connections. In contrast to the literal-minded Sensor, the Intuitive doesn't take statements at face value but automatically makes a figurative interpretation. Don't expect a lot of explanation—Intuitives just assume that you will make the appropriate connections and fill in the gaps as their own minds flit from one association to another.

> I am not one of those who in expressing opinions confine themselves to facts.
>
> MARK TWAIN

Intuitives are not especially interested in discussing factual or concrete matters—weather, transportation, the cost of living, and the like. When reading, they scan passages to get the overall meaning; both on the page and in reality, they spend little time on details or facts, which can appear too obvious to them to merit very much attention.

Intuitives tend to read between the lines, listening for and finding or creating underlying meanings in other people's words. Sensitive to the subtleties, nuances, and implications in communication, they are attuned to a person's body language, facial expression, and vocal inflections. When watching the characters in a movie, they take all of these factors into account and automatically interpret the characters' behavior; it would never even occur to them to take what a character says at face value. The same is true in real life.

Romance with the Intuitive

Intuitives tend to be romantic in their ideas about love and may spend years searching for an ideal partner. At first blush, *most* possible partners appear to be "the one." In the Intuitive's mind (which, as you probably know by now, is where all the action really takes place), a date begins as soon as the plans for it are made. Instantly, Intuitives project an idealized vision onto Ms. or Mr. Friday Night Date and then become increasingly caught up in the fantasy of this perfect potential partner. Needless to say, reality rarely lives up to their expectations, especially for Intuitives who are also Feelers. Thinkers tend to be more realistic.

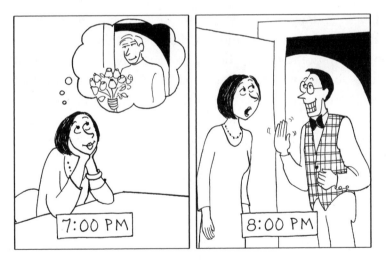

7:00 PM   8:00 PM

A night out on the town is not the Intuitive's idea of a great date. Unlike Sensors, Intuitives tend to be indifferent to traditional forms of entertainment and see little appeal in a relationship that revolves around nightclubs, sporting events, box-office hits, and the like. A stimulating conversation in almost any setting, on the other hand, is always a turn-on.

Once involved with a romantic partner, the Intuitive views the relationship as an opportunity for growth and learning. Change and improvement are vital to keep a connection alive. Intuitives often thrive in relationships with other Intuitives, who share their strong need for a mental connection. Sparks may fly in the bedroom, but an Intuitive couple really bonds through intimate discussions about philosophy and the deeper meanings of life.

Intuitives at Work

Discovery consists of seeing what everybody has seen and thinking what nobody has thought.

ALBERT VON SZENT-GYORGYI

Intuitives are drawn to work that requires insight and imagination—qualities they possess in abundance. Because Intuitives are so strongly oriented toward the future, they often have original and unusual perceptions about emerging trends and needs. Resourceful in solving problems and creating new ways of doing things, the Intuitive finds innovation exciting and usually feels stifled when required to take a traditional by-the-book approach. Making innovative or creative leaps is the Intuitive's strong suit, not systematically applying past experience, existing knowledge, or empirical proof.

The Pilgrims didn't have any experience when they landed here. Hell, if experience was that important, we'd never have anybody walking on the moon.

DOUG RADER

Intuitives are not content to just "make a living." It's possible for an Intuitive to leave a job interview without ever having inquired about the salary. Although circumstances may lead an Intuitive to take a less compelling job, it is very important to most of them that the work be personally meaningful. They may find certain positions appealing because they share the values of the organization, or because the work offers an opportunity to make a positive change in the world or to brainstorm with other creative people. Independent and inherently suspicious of authority, they don't think twice about flouting rules that are not compatible with their own values. Working in a traditional, structured organization, such as a government or military environment, is not usually very appealing to an Intuitive.

Working with those who share similar values, the Intuitive can make a strong teammate or persuasive leader, inspiring ingenuity in others and helping them push past what is merely accepted or expected. Intuitives are often more talented at thinking things up than they are at executing them or making them work. When the main problems are solved and the initial challenge wears off, they can lose interest and become bored. That's why it's good for an Intuitive to partner with a Sensor at work.

More than practical, down-to-earth Sensors, Intuitives can have visions that are difficult to implement. Because Intuitives tend to have high expectations of themselves, they can become discouraged when they fall short of their goals. And since their ideas can change rapidly, the final concept may bear only a vague resemblance to the original.

Famous Intuitives

Barack Obama, Stephen Hawking, Alice Walker,
Alice Miller, Shirley MacLaine, Oprah Winfrey,
Robin Williams, Mohandas Gandhi, Susan B. Anthony,
Michael Moore, Bill Maher, Jon Stewart,
Carl Jung, Sigmund Freud

> If you can dream it, you can do it. Always remember that this whole thing was started with a dream and a mouse.
>
> WALT DISNEY

> I shut my eyes in order to see.
>
> PAUL GAUGUIN

> Intuition is the clear concept of the whole at once.
>
> RALPH WALDO EMERSON

What Drives an Intuitive Crazy

• Blow-by-blow descriptions

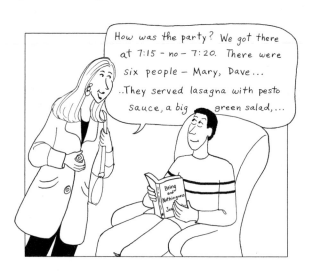

> Reporting facts is the refuge of those
> who have no imagination.
>
> LUC, MARQUIS DE VAUVENARGUES

- Tedious or mundane tasks

- Pragmatists who insist on poking holes in other people's ideas

- People who can't see beyond the obvious and seem oblivious to deeper meanings

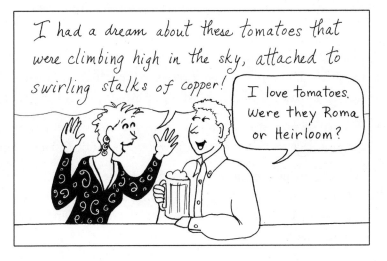

- People who don't understand that it's okay to differ from the norm

- People who have no imagination

- Insignificant details

> Talk to him of Jacob's ladder, and he
> would ask the number of the steps.
>
> DOUGLAS WILLIAM JERROLD

81

- Knowing there's a better way to do something—but being the only one who cares

I'm an Intuitive. Now What?

- Find a balance between focusing on your ideals and visions and attending to the details of everyday reality. Turn off your "possibility generator" some of the time, or at least try to understand how some people might find it tiring.

- When starting a project, consider what will actually be required. Even if it's tedious, factor in all the details in order to estimate how long it will take. Leave extra time for the unforeseen.

- Seek out places where you're likely to encounter other Intuitives, such as classes or events that revolve around literature, metaphysics, psychology, or spirituality. It feeds your soul to interact with others who perceive the world as you do.

- Practice keeping your attention on the present moment and gently escort it back to the here and now when you notice it wandering.

- When sharing a brand-new idea, avoid potential embarrassment—and wasting the time and energy of others—by letting people know that you're nowhere near ready to implement it yet.

- Allow others to give you feedback on the feasibility and possible pitfalls of your ideas. Sometimes they will be right, and even if they're not, you still get points for being open to suggestions.

- We all have a deep need for others to "get" us, so take the time to present your ideas simply and clearly if you want them to be more widely understood and accepted.

Be obscure clearly.

E. B. WHITE

- Complexity may be seductive to you, but allow yourself to do some things the simple or ordinary way.

A soul occupied with great ideas
performs small duties.

HARRIET MARTINEAU

- The next time you're itching for a change, go for a moderate refinement, not a big sweeping improvement.

- Accept some things as they are; not everything must be made over according to your ideal.

Idealism is fine, but as it approaches
reality the cost becomes prohibitive.

WILLIAM F. BUCKLEY JR.

- Pay attention to the simple joys of everyday life. Take time to stop, look, listen, smell, feel, and taste. Let your senses become overloaded once in a while. Unplug!

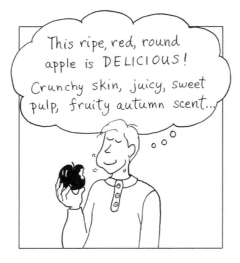

- If you have young children in your life, take note of their here-and-now approach to the world. Usually, you'll find them completely caught up in the moment, absolutely absorbed in watching a caterpillar on the sidewalk, blowing bubbles in the bath, or feeling the sand sliding through their fingers.

- Respect your need for time to dream, fantasize, read, and create (though not, perhaps, while on the clock at your job).

So you see, imagination needs
moodling—long, inefficient, happy
idling, dawdling and uttering.

BRENDA UELAND

6

The Sensor/Intuitive Relationship

Of all the four preference pairs, Sensors and Intuitives will experience differences that are perhaps the most important to recognize, understand, and honor in intimate or romantic relationships. Sensing and intuition determine how we communicate on a day-to-day basis. Since good communication is so important to a healthy relationship, couples with the same preference on this dimension have a big advantage over those who do not. That doesn't mean that there are no successful Sensor/Intuitive pairings, but such couples usually have to work harder to understand each other.

To the outside observer, it can look like the two members of a Sensor/Intuitive couple come from different planets and have little common ground on which to base a relationship. And in fact, it can seem that way to the couple themselves. Yet there's no doubt that Sensors and Intuitives can be drawn to each other. The pragmatic, down-to-earth Sensor often admires the ingenuity, innovativeness, and creativity of the Intuitive. The different approach can seem quite alluring to the Sensor, who usually finds it easier to adapt to an opposite-preference partner than the Intuitive does. But Intuitives can be perplexing to Sensors too, with their abstract, complex communication style. They seem more complicated—and they are!

Intuitives, for their part, often appreciate the Sensor's interest in the practical matters of life. The Sensor can provide solid ground beneath the Intuitive's feet and help him or her be more present in—and more comfortable with—everyday reality. But in the company of a Sensor, an Intuitive may sense the absence of some vital connection between them.

The biggest problem a Sensor/Intuitive couple usually faces is an inability to understand or appreciate each other's communication style. What is said, meant, or heard can be perceived very differently by each of the parties. In short order, this difference in perception ceases to seem interesting or amusing and simply becomes a pain in the posterior. The beginning of a relationship, when the attraction is strongest and the motivation to get along is highest, is the ideal time for the couple to study their differences and learn how to work with (or around) them, but it's never too late to improve the situation. After all, sensing and intuition are natural preferences, not choices we deliberately make to drive each other crazy.

In a couple composed of two Sensors, by way of contrast, there is a great deal of common ground. They don't have to wonder whether they're misinterpreting each other; they understand each other's literal communication style. Both share a realistic, practical view of the world. Both take life at face value, enjoying the here and now without getting hung up on what it may—or may not—all mean. And both may share many interests, depending on how their three other preferences line up. All this is good news for romance—since 75 to 85 percent of the general population are Sensors, the odds are high that both parties in any given couple will in fact be Sensors. On the downside—and of course there is *always* a downside—two Sensors can become stuck in their ways when their intuitive sides are not developed. Under stress, they may fall into "catastrophe mode," both thinking of all the things that could go wrong.

Two Intuitives are very likely to communicate well as a couple, depending on how their other three preferences match up. Both are stimulated by lively discussion about new ideas and exciting possibilities, and both are quick to grasp underlying meanings. Both live more fully in their minds than in their bodies, and each appreciates a partner who accepts this as normal. On the downside, dealing with routine and mundane tasks can be challenging, especially if both are strong Intuitives. By default, everyday chores (such as paying the bills, housecleaning, grocery shopping, and cooking) usually fall to the partner who is either more moderate on this preference scale or somewhat less averse to doing them—often the woman.

Still, the opposite-preference couple is the most likely to face the greatest challenges. This does not mean that they cannot have a happy, successful relationship (especially if their three other preferences are the same), but they must be able to acknowledge the validity of different ways of seeing the world. When each partner feels that his or her way of perceiving is understood and appreciated by the other, the two of them can complement each other, bringing balance to the relationship instead of conflict. And because the combined perceptions of sensing and intuition are always more accurate and complete than those of the individual components in this kind of "mixed" relationship, the two parties can benefit from listening to each other's views. On the other hand, it is certainly far less challenging if they are not too far apart on this dimension. It is often couples with more moderate preferences on this dimension who find it easier to understand each other than do those who have a strong preference.

Here are several techniques that I have found effective in improving communication, decreasing stress, and increasing respect between opposite-preference partners.

How to Get Along with a Sensor

- Compliment the Sensor on his or her common sense and appreciate your partner's ability to be present, right here, right now.

- Try to participate in the Sensor's sense-oriented world: create a feast together, plant a garden, go skiing, sailing, or river rafting. Attend a sporting event together, or a music festival.

- Join the Sensor for the holiday celebrations that are important to him or her.

- Be patient when the Sensor talks about specifics and details.

- If you want your ideas to be accepted by a Sensor, stress their feasibility, usefulness, and practical application. Sensors need to be convinced that something will work. Keep in mind that errors of fact will destroy your credibility.

- When a Sensor asks you a specific question, give a specific answer.

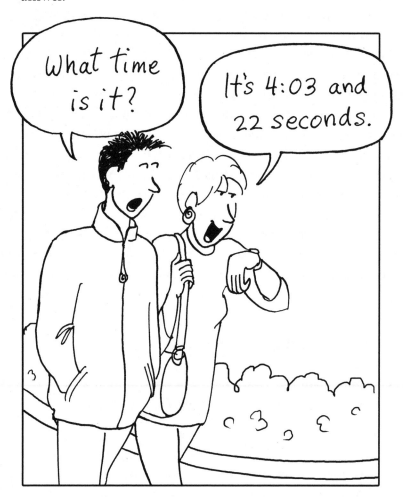

- Appreciate the Sensor for the tangible, day-to-day ways—making meals, washing the car, mowing the lawn, fixing things—in which this person makes life more comfortable for you. Do practical things for the Sensor in return.

> The four most important words in any
> marriage: "I'll do the dishes."
>
> ANONYMOUS

- To make your ideas better understood and accepted, present them simply, clearly, and precisely. Simplify rather than complicate your communications. Avoid vague or abstract explanations. Use familiar terms. Give real examples to make your point.

- Provide the Sensor with sensory stimulation—back rubs, massages, lovemaking.

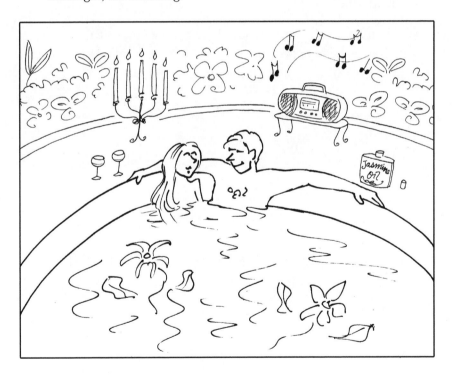

- Keep in mind that satisfying experiences for Sensors involve things they can see, touch, hear, smell, and taste.

Statements That Sensors Hate to Hear

"Don't be a stick in the mud."
"Boring, boring, boring."
"Enough with the details."
"Can't you see beyond the obvious?"
"Use your imagination."
"Do you always have to do it the same way?"

How to Get Along with an Intuitive

- Don't give an Intuitive all the details of your day. Learn to share the highlights.

- When an Intuitive discusses his or her ideas, give this person a chance to share the "big picture." Postpone addressing what may seem unrealistic or impractical to you.

You see things and you say, Why?·But I dream
things that never were and I say, Why not?

GEORGE BERNARD SHAW

- Don't expect Intuitives to follow through on all their ideas. They often just enjoy coming up with them . . . and that's all they need to do to feel satisfied.

· The best way to have a good idea
is to have lots of ideas.

LINUS PAULING

- Whenever possible, the Intuitive likes to focus on the more creative and inventive aspects of a project. He or she is happiest when others work out the bugs and handle the details. If you yourself enjoy working on the nitty-gritty, offer help.

- Be especially mindful to not nitpick with an Intuitive about the details and specifics.

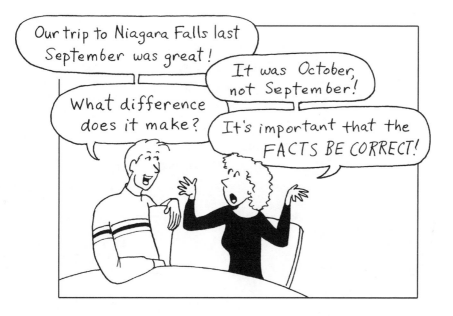

- Keep in mind that Intuitives may rebel and not even bother to complete a task when the boundaries are too clearly defined.

- Spend time fantasizing about future possibilities with an Intuitive. Have fun making wish lists together of desired trips, purchases, and the like. Even though your dreams may never become reality, enjoy the process. Don't take the wind out of your Intuitive's sails by pointing out what or why something won't work.

- Transactions outside the bedroom can be a turn-on. Ideas arouse an Intuitive's mind as well as his or her body.

- Compliment your Intuitive partner on his or her innovative and creative problem-solving skills or abilities.

- Seek an Intuitive's advice about alternative solutions to problems when your usual way isn't working.

- Be patient with an Intuitive's sometimes complicated way of describing things. If it's hard for you to follow or understand, ask questions.

Statements That Intuitives Hate to Hear

"Your head is _always_ in the clouds." ✓

"You're a dreamer." ≈

"Be more realistic." ✓

"You're not being practical."

"Come down to earth." ✓

"What's wrong with it the way it is?"

"You're always off in the future."

7

The Decision-Making Preference

THINKERS/FEELERS

Read the following statements and check the sentence that describes you best—A or B. To achieve the most accurate score, answer the statements according to what is true for you, not according to what you would like to be true or think ought to be true. Be mindful of the pressure in our society for men to be logical, rational, and analytical (Thinkers) and for women to be warm, nurturing, and supportive (Feelers).

The Inventory

1. A ☐ People would probably describe me as detached and impersonal.
   B ☒ People would probably describe me as warm and supportive.

2. A ☐ I value my ability to be rational.
   B ☒ I value my ability to be empathetic.

3. A ☐ I enjoy debating and defending my point of view.
   B ☒ I dislike arguing and debating. I value harmony.

4. A ☐ I make decisions objectively and impersonally.

   B ☒ I make decisions based on how other people will be affected.

5. A ☐ It is more important to be truthful than tactful.

   B ☒ It is more important to be tactful than truthful.

6. A ☐ I tend to pay more attention to people's thoughts than their feelings.

   B ☒ I tend to pay more attention to people's feelings than their thoughts.

7. A ☐ I am good at critiquing people.

   B ☒ I am good at appreciating people.

8. A ☐ I tend to analyze people's problems.

   B ☒ I tend to sympathize with people's problems.

9. A ☐ I tend to not take remarks personally.

   B ☒ My feelings are easily hurt.

10. A ☐ I make decisions based primarily on principles of justice and fairness.

    B ☒ I make decisions based primarily on personal circumstances or concerns.

Scoring

In the first blank space below, record how many times you chose A as the answer to one of the questions. In the second blank space below, record how many times you chose B.

Total

___0___ A   Thinker
___10___ B   Feeler

Thinkers and Feelers in a Nutshell

This third set of opposites refers to how people evaluate information, make decisions, and arrive at conclusions. Thinkers make decisions based on a rational, logical, analytical process. Striving to be impartial, they place more value on consistency and fairness than on how others will respond to their decisions.

Feelers, on the other hand, make decisions more subjectively, based on a personal value system that takes into account how they and others will be affected, what is best for all involved, and the goal of creating or maintaining harmony. Just as the Thinker does, a Feeler will consider objective arguments, but he or she doesn't place undue emphasis on them or view consistency and fairness as top priorities.

It's important to keep in mind that although a Thinker's feelings are not always visible, Thinkers do *have* feelings. Conversely, although Feelers may not always verbalize their logic, the Feeler is completely capable of logical thought. Note that "thinking," as the term is used in the Myers-Briggs system of personality assessment, refers only to how an individual makes decisions, not to their degree of intellectual development. The term "feeling" addresses the decision-making process as well, not the depth of emotion.

Although we all make some decisions entirely by a thinking process and other decisions entirely by a feeling process, most decisions involve both. Each of us, then, no matter what type we are, functions in the thinking realm as well as in the feeling realm—but each of us also puts more trust in one realm than in the other. For all of us, the decisions we find the most difficult are those in which the thinking side conflicts with the feeling side. In that situation, our preference usually takes over. Similarly, a decision that we make easily and that we feel good about is usually one in which our feeling and thinking sides are in sync with each other. Using both preferences is also useful when you're completely unsure of how to proceed in a given situation. First try making your decision based on your preference. Then make the decision again using the opposite preference—and notice what you failed to take into account the first time around. With this more complete picture in mind, you will be better able to make a thoughtful final decision.

Some people find it difficult to determine whether they have a stronger preference for thinking or feeling because their natural tendency may go against their conditioning, especially if it is along gender lines. Thinking-Feeling is the only set of opposites in which there is a gender difference. In most cultures, women are socialized to behave like Feelers—to be sensitive, tactful, and nurturing and to choose traditional female careers such as nursing or teaching. Men are socialized to behave like Thinkers—to be logical, objective, competitive, direct, and assertive and to pursue traditional male careers such as engineering, law, or accounting. Not surprisingly, then, about 65 to 75 percent of Thinkers are male, while 25 to 35 percent are female. This means, of course, that 65 to 75 percent of Feelers are female, while 25 to 35 percent are male.

To what extent these statistics reflect a tendency to provide the "right" answer to inventory questions is unknown. But it is clear that females who have a natural preference for thinking and males who have a natural preference for feeling are in the minority. Being in the minority can sometimes make these men and women feel unaccepted, out of sync, or distressingly different from how they think they should be. The reactions they receive from others tend to reinforce a sense of alienation. Females with a strong preference for thinking are sometimes perceived as cold, uncaring, and aggressive, while males who have a strong preference for feeling can be seen as too soft and "feminine." To fit in and feel accepted, these men and women learn to adapt their behavior, sometimes even coming to mistrust their natural way of making decisions.

It is easier to be a thinking female or a feeling male today than in the past, but the challenges still exist, and they can have a significant impact on a person's self-esteem. As society encourages and educates men to be more aware of their feelings and women to feel more comfortable with their analytical abilities, this unhealthy dynamic may change.

THINKERS

You Might Be a Thinker If . . .

- You don't usually get described as "warm and fuzzy." "Cold and abrupt" is more like it.

- You'd rather play chess than go to a spirituality seminar.

- Critiquing the ideas of others is second nature.

- Writing mushy love notes is not one of your fortes.

- You'd rather see an adventure or mystery film than a romantic drama.

- You're unlikely to lose sleep after firing an employee . . . or before!

- You've considered auditioning for *Jeopardy!*

- You turn up the volume when discussions on scientific or economic topics come on the radio.

- You're allergic to the idea of therapy. Your personal life is nobody's business but your own.

Thinkers at Their Best	Thinkers at Their Worst
Objective	Critical
Rational	Abrupt
Competent	Impersonal
Analytical	Stubborn
Levelheaded	Intellectually arrogant
Intellectually stimulating	Skeptical
Authoritative	Dismissive
Cognitive	Insensitive

Thinkers 101

I exist because I think.

JEAN-PAUL SARTRE

Thinkers prefer to make decisions in an impersonal or impartial way, based on logic and analysis. They pride themselves on their ability to remain objective and levelheaded. To assess and determine the best course of action and to make a reasonable and rational decision, a Thinker uses cause-and-effect reasoning, weighing and comparing information against a basic set of criteria. Thinkers like to analyze and examine the pros and cons, ramifications, and consequences of decisions. They place more value on consistency than on how their decisions will affect others. Because they want to be fair, the rules that apply to one situation must also apply to another. They are not as interested in the personal circumstances that may be involved. In order to keep their personal bias out of the decision-making process, Thinkers put feelings aside. Emotions, including their own, are no more than data to consider. Subjective evaluations of a situation seem unreliable, and to a Thinker, feelings are not something to rely on.

Feelings are untidy.

ESTHER HAUTZIG

Although Thinkers can and do care deeply about people and issues, their decisions are rarely based solely on their personal feelings. As a result, they're able to make decisions, even difficult ones, fairly easily. Their decisiveness and aura of confidence can be quite attractive to some people, but these same qualities make them look cold and detached to others (especially to Feelers.)

Communicating with a Thinker

For Thinkers, communication is an opportunity to impart or receive information, not necessarily to commune or bond. Interactions with a Thinker tend to focus on a specific objective. In discussions, Thinkers prefer that the communication stay focused on the topic at hand, which they're good at following. When others discuss personal matters, Thinkers sometimes become impatient or abrupt.

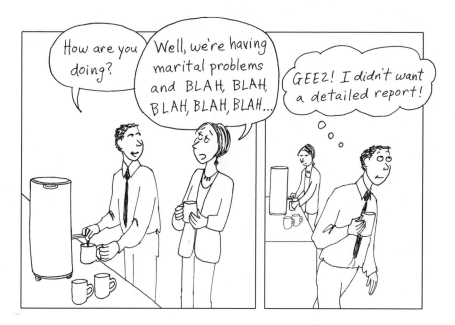

When communicating with a Thinker, you're likely to hear statements such as:

"Let's look at the pros and cons."

"I'll keep this brief."

"That's not logical."

"We need to be objective about the situation."

Direct and straightforward, Thinkers often have strong opinions or convictions that they don't hesitate to express. And they can go to great lengths to prove that they're right. In the minds of Thinkers, honesty is the best policy, so when they disagree with someone they'll say so, even at the risk of offending the person. Because they value truth more than tact, they can easily say the wrong thing at the wrong time and end up clashing with others. Since they themselves tend to not take remarks personally, they often assume that other people won't be upset by their comments.

Debating and competitive banter offer Thinkers a no-risk situation: either they'll prevail or they'll learn something new. They win either way. Thinkers like to argue for fun or sport once in a while. They respect others who can defend a different view. A good fight can be exciting, and they often take an opposing stance just for the heck of it. In the Thinkers' world, disagreements may be momentarily stressful, but most skirmishes . . . at least in small doses . . . end up being productive in the long run.

> Too much agreement kills a chat.
>
> ELDRIDGE CLEAVER

When a conflict involves personal issues about a relationship, however, the Thinker is apt to shy away.

Relating Intimately with a Thinker

Thinkers are not likely to be "touchy-feely" types. In their attempts to understand love by analyzing, scrutinizing, and dissecting it, their objective analysis can be perceived as impersonal or uncaring—especially by a Feeling partner or would-be partner. Thinkers do not bring as much intensity to intimacy as Feelers do, and in fact, keeping up with the emotional intensity of a Feeler can be challenging for them. Frequent reassurances of love and caring are not usually forthcoming from Thinkers.

Although this sounds like a contradiction in terms, Thinkers are capable of a detached intimacy. They are likely to view sex from a merely physical perspective rather than as an opportunity for expressing affection, but because they are always trying to improve at everything, including sex, they can be enthusiastic and passionate lovers. They are certainly capable of feeling overpowering love, but expressing it adequately or appropriately is challenging. When Thinkers recognize the emotional needs of those close to them, they can be supportive and attentive, making an honest effort to meet those needs. If a healthy relationship is their goal, they'll do everything they can to foster and maintain it.

Given the difficulty that Thinkers can have expressing warmth, tenderness, and caring, you'd never guess how deep their affections sometimes run. They're more comfortable expressing their fondness for friends and loved ones, not with words, but through actions: fixing things, solving problems, offering advice. It's important to notice the things that Thinkers do that demonstrate caring.

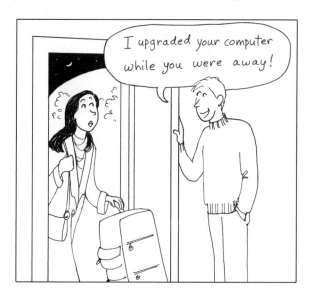

It can be challenging for Thinkers to feel their emotions, both positive and negative. A Thinker's emotions originate in his or her head as abstract thoughts, and they move to the heart only after thorough analysis. The more Thinkers understand their emotions, the freer they are to experience or express them. Although Thinkers tend to manage their outer lives competently, the inner landscape can look relatively barren.

The intellectual defenses of Thinkers don't allow them to expose their emotional concerns until they really trust someone. When a topic touches on emotional issues, they can be poor communicators, responding with logic and reason rather than empathetic support. They are likely to postpone dealing with unwieldy concerns about feelings or to manage them with curt dismissals.

A typical Thinker's modus operandi is to act as though everything is okay, meanwhile holding so much inside that high stress levels can develop. As a result, bottled-up emotions sometimes erupt unexpectedly, much to everyone's surprise, including the Thinker's. This internal dynamic can create an unhappy cycle: to avoid any more embarrassing expressions of vulnerability, Thinkers may redouble their efforts to conceal their feelings.

Because Thinkers are not naturally empathetic, placing themselves in another person's shoes and understanding needs that differ from their own can be difficult. Because they tend to minimize the emotional aspects of communications coming from others, they're sometimes accused of being insensitive. Most of the time, however, they are puzzled by this response and cannot understand why others are angry or upset with them.

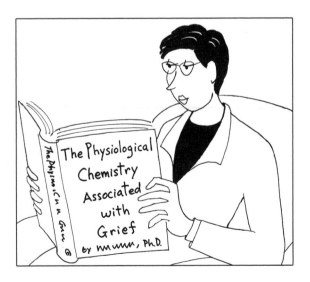

Although Thinkers seem to be impervious to the opinions of others, they can actually be as sensitive as anyone else to rejection or criticism. This vulnerable side is hidden by a show of coolness and detachment, however, sometimes without the Thinker even being aware of it.

Thinkers at Work

Thinkers gravitate toward work that appeals to their ability to analyze problems logically and make objective decisions. They enjoy working with colleagues who are just as competent, skilled, and reasonable as they are. If they don't respect a colleague's abilities, they have difficulty trusting that person. Thinkers find employment easily since, in most organizations, thinking is the accepted mode of decision-making. They tend to do well in their jobs or careers. For them, money is a measure of success and enables them to exercise power and control.

Because Thinkers have high expectations of themselves, learning a new skill can be frustrating until they're able to perform up to their standards. Once they've achieved this comfort level, they enjoy the challenge of solving problems, the tougher the better. Thinkers are good at analyzing and assessing objectives, setting priorities and goals, and organizing facts or ideas into logical sequences. They're also adept at identifying what is inconsistent, inefficient, or illogical.

Thinkers tend to define their success and happiness by what they *do* in the world. Their self-esteem comes from being capable and competent and accomplishing the things they set their minds to do. Partly because they themselves are capable of high achievement and partly because they lack empathy for those in different circumstances, Thinkers believe that everyone can make something of themselves if they just work hard enough.

Since they fully expect everyone to perform competently (including themselves), Thinkers seldom see the need to congratulate or praise anyone for a job well done. On the other hand, they can be quick to tell others where they need to improve.

Thinkers tend to form and rely on their own opinions independent of the reactions of others. They're also more capable of developing an independent image of their self-worth and to determine when they've done something well.

Famous Thinkers

Al Gore, Dick Cheney, Hillary Clinton, Dave Letterman, Jay Leno, Michael Jordan, Newt Gingrich, Bill O'Reilly, Maria Shriver, Mike Wallace, Ted Koppel, Joan Rivers, Jon Stewart, Alan Greenspan, Clint Eastwood, Joy Behar

> We should take care not to make the intellect our god; it has, of course, powerful muscles, but no personality.
>
> ALBERT EINSTEIN

What Drives a Thinker Crazy

- Illogical thinking

- Too much talk about feelings

- Exaggerated praise

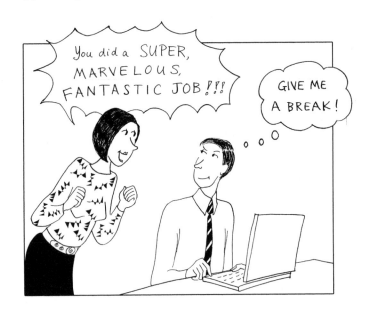

- People who can't take criticism

- People who bring their personal problems to work

- Being asked to bend the rules or make exceptions

- Being asked to provide emotional reassurance

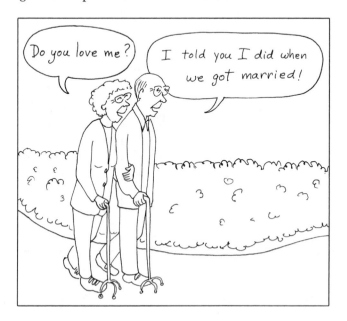

- Public displays of affection

I'm a Thinker. Now What?

- Recognize the limits of rational thinking and cerebral understanding. Thinking is a vital tool in the impersonal realm; you wouldn't be able to write up a contract, program a computer, build a deck, or perform myriad other useful activities without it. As you may have noticed, however, the impersonal approach is less successful when it comes to dealing with people.

- When others bring up their personal problems, avoid analyzing or trying to fix them. Not every problem needs to be solved. Many times people just want to be heard or understood.

- Make an extra effort to express appreciation to others, even for the small things they do. Instead of pointing out what needs correcting, mention what is well done.

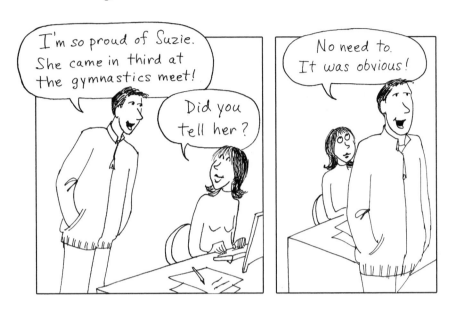

- Practice being more self-revealing with the people you trust.

- In a discussion or argument, really listen to the other person's point of view and try to see things from a different perspective.

- Refrain from telling others what they should or shouldn't do. No matter how certain you are that you are right, remember that such pronouncements usually result in hurt feelings and resentment.

- Expand your sense of self to include more than what you do or what you achieve.

- Avoid being so analytical in a dispute that you miss the emotional aspect of what's going on. Logic often has little to do with the feelings involved.

- Watch your tendency to play the devil's advocate. Don't intimidate to win an argument or get your way.

- Beware of overwhelming others with your bluntness or directness. If you happen to hurt someone's feelings with a thoughtless remark, apologize sincerely and resolve to be more mindful next time.

Words once spoken can never be recalled.

WENTWORTH DILLON

To handle yourself, use your head; to handle others, use your heart.

ANONYMOUS

Female Thinkers

Men in Western cultures are socialized to be logical, rational, independent, straightforward, and direct—all inherent traits, you might recall, of the Thinking preference. But female Thinkers are less accepted because these traits are seen as "masculine." Not only can the clash between personality and cultural expectations cause an inner struggle for them, but it can also create barriers to satisfying relationships with men or friendships with feeling-type women. Thinker girls usually learn to soften their style, however, because they grow up hearing that "real" women are nurturing, sensitive, and compassionate. Their feelings can become developed and refined through serving as the primary caregiver of their children and providing support to their partner. Still, female Thinkers often have less need to nurture and take care of others than do more traditional feeling-type women. And because people tend to fall back on their natural or trusted style in conflict situations women Thinkers are capable of being tough or aggressive. As a result, they can have access to the best of both worlds—objectivity and subjectivity, reason and compassion.

You Might Be a Feeler If . . .

Depends
- The words "Don't take it personally" make you take that remark *really* personally.

- You would refuse a high-paying job in the Housing Eviction Department.

- You need a box of tissues to get through a Hallmark commercial.

✓ • Praising others is second nature.

✓ • You refuse to see a violent movie.

✓ • You're the one who is most likely to buy the get-well card for one of your co-workers and personally deliver it, along with a bouquet from your garden, a vat of chicken soup, and your promise to check in every day until she's back on her feet.

✓ • You are both touchy and feely.

✓ • You worry about whether your neighbor's dog gets enough attention.

✓ • Your friend said to buy the fuel-efficient car, but you went for the sky-blue gas guzzler because you loved the color.

✓ • When you think you've upset someone, you call right away to apologize . . . and then call again to re-apologize.

Feelers at Their Best	Feelers at Their Worst
Warm	Too emotional
Sympathetic	Thin-skinned and overly sensitive
Helpful	Overly accommodating
Kind	Too subjective
Thoughtful	Unassertive
Tactful	Indirect
Cooperative	Manipulative
Sensitive	Hysterical

Feelers 101

> It is wisdom to believe the heart.
>
> GEORGE SANTAYANA

Feelers make decisions according to their personal values rather than objective criteria as Thinkers do. Primarily, they consider how their actions will affect others and make decisions subjectively, based on what they believe is right according to their personal values. Feelers are good at such assessments. But because they allow for extenuating circumstances and are always concerned about others, the decision-making process can prove challenging for them, especially when the decision might affect someone adversely. Feelers consider objective arguments, but they don't place undue emphasis on them. When logic contradicts their values, they respond by ignoring or undervaluing it. When Feelers try to be objective, they believe that they're overlooking something crucial—the personal values that really matter to themselves and others.

> Better to be without logic than without feeling.
>
> CHARLOTTE BRONTË

Communicating with a Feeler

Feelers perceive communication as an opportunity to interact and connect with others, not merely as a way to exchange information. In fact, they find Thinker-style exchanges that focus primarily on content unsatisfying. For the Feeler, genuine communication is about openness, sharing, empathy, and emotional responses. In conversation and correspondence, they focus mainly on relationships and the ins and outs of interpersonal dynamics, personal and meaningful happenings, and the values that matter deeply to them. Feelers usually display less interest in discussing impersonal matters such as business, sports, or research.

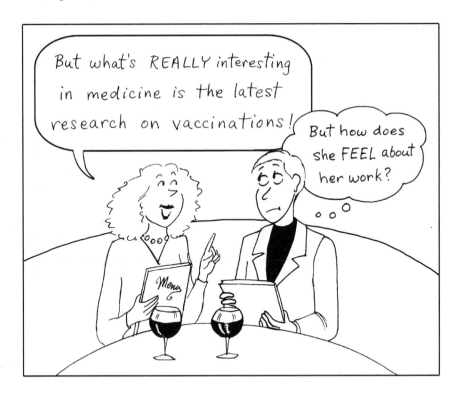

In discussions or when teaching or presenting information, Feelers often use anecdotes or human interest stories to put a warmer, more personal spin on the material. Not only do they want people to like what they have to say, but they very much want to be liked themselves. Feelers find it particularly painful when others regard them with antipathy, or even when others are simply indifferent.

I have a fear of being disliked, even by people I dislike.

OPRAH WINFREY

In conversation with a Feeler, you're likely to hear statements along these lines:

"I appreciate your help."

"That really matters to me."

"Sue is feeling a bit under the weather. It would make me happy if you'd call her."

"I feel that Johnny is sincerely trying to do better at school."

To avoid an unpleasant exchange that might undermine a relationship, a Feeler will try to redirect the conversation to a more positive topic or will skirt an issue to avoid disappointing, displeasing, or hurting the other person. When especially concerned about alienating another, Feelers might even take back a statement they've already uttered or act as though they agree with the other person's position. These surprising about-faces stem in part from a desire to end the conflict, but also from the Feeler's ability to see another's point of view and empathize with it. You won't find Feelers switching sides, however, on issues they care deeply about. They're passionate about the things that really matter to them, and when their values are threatened, they don't hesitate to stand up for their rights and for those of others as well.

Relating Intimately with a Feeler

For Feelers, love is a matter of the heart. Intimacy is an opportunity to express love and caring. Love is something that is felt, not something to be analyzed, dissected, scrutinized, objectified, or improved upon, as it can be for Thinkers.

Oh you who are trying to learn the marvel of Love through the copy book of reason, I'm very much afraid that you will never really see the point.

ḤĀFEZ OF SHIRAZ

Because relationships are of paramount importance to Feelers, they strive to maintain close connections with those they care about. To a friend in emotional pain, there's no more comforting shoulder to cry on than that of a Feeler. The Feeler focuses on the potential good in each person and takes an interest in their welfare. Feelers are good listeners—understanding, sympathetic, and perceptive about what's going on with others. People are often drawn to Feelers when they need support.

In the typical Feeler's value system, being tactful is more important than telling the "cold" truth. If they absolutely must confront someone or express disagreement or disappointment, they'll handle the situation as diplomatically as possible. As a result, giving negative feedback, even when well deserved, can be as problematic for the Feeler as receiving it. Because their feelings are easily hurt, Feelers tend to assume that other people are equally sensitive. When criticized, they can withdraw, become insecure, and lose confidence. Some can become irrational and emotional and will see the criticism as an indictment of their character.

Although others are sometimes impatient or uncomfortable with the Feeler's emotions, it's best to avoid suggesting that they're being overly sensitive or irrational. When stressed or upset, Feelers recover more quickly if they don't try to quash their emotions. Once they've had the opportunity to experience their feelings, they are able to see things in a more objective light. When they share how they're feeling, they like to be met with empathy and not have you try to solve their problems or point out what you'd do in their place, unless they ask for it.

Feelers have the tendency to idealize the people they admire. They can have a hard time seeing and accepting a difficult truth about someone they care about and can overlook the person's negative points. They can also hang on to inappropriate relationships for too long, or they may take on the responsibility for the failure of a relationship.

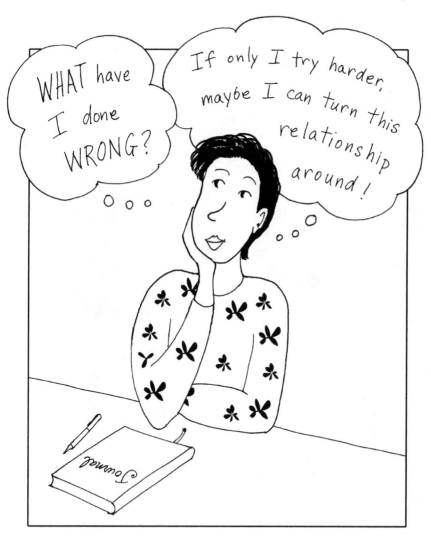

Some Feelers become overly involved in the lives of others, so much so that they risk losing a sense of themselves. And because of their deep need for approval, it's not uncommon for Feelers to exhibit chameleon-like behavior as they try to change themselves to be more pleasing to the person they are with.

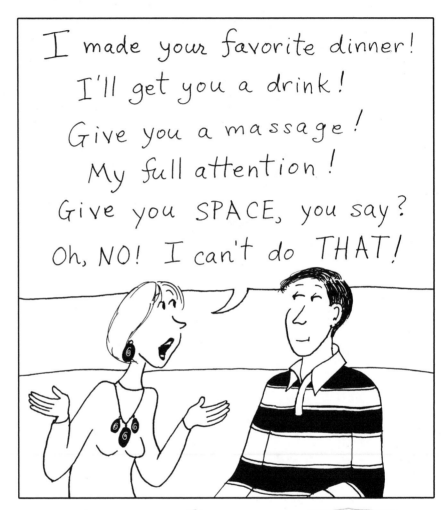

Ironically, Feelers can be better friends to others than they are to themselves. Often they struggle to value their own needs and desires appropriately. Some Feelers put other people's needs before their own, with the sometimes tragic result that they sacrifice their own needs, interests, or goals in the process. Because Feelers tend to be accommodating, others can take advantage of them, possibly causing them to feel resentful. Feelers may find themselves in an unhealthy, unbalanced relationship.

Feelers at Work

*When people go to work, they shouldn't
have to leave their hearts at home.*

BETTY BENDER

Feelers enjoy working in congenial, supportive environments where
they are valued and respected not just for their skills or knowledge but
for who they are. They perform best when their colleagues like and
appreciate them and listen to their ideas and points of view. Working with people who don't encourage and affirm them presents a
major challenge for approval-seeking Feelers, since they don't usually
have the detachment (as Thinkers do) to evaluate their self-worth
independently.

A contentious or competitive work environment poses another
workplace hazard. Not only does conflict cause psychological discomfort to the Feeler, but sometimes it even leads to emotional or physical illness. And work that is impersonal can be a turnoff, unless it
has some strong underlying meaning for the Feeler. When both the
work environment and the work itself reflect their personal values and
contribute to something they care deeply about, Feelers can be highly
motivated. They are loyal and devoted to persons, institutions, and
causes they believe in.

Idealism is both a blessing and a curse for the Feeler. On the plus
side, Feelers strive to create greater goodwill in the world, and many
of our great activists and healers have been Feelers (Mother Teresa,
Martin Luther King Jr., Florence Nightingale). On the downside, some
Feelers are deeply affected by interpersonal tensions and can become
quite anxious or upset in the face of conflict, especially if their efforts
to improve the situation fail. Feelers have faith that equilibrium can
be restored—and in fact they often manage to bring that about.

Feelers are capable of handling money (and they certainly can and
do), but their attitude toward it can be ambivalent. To the Feeler's way
of thinking, money is secondary to human needs and is too often

linked to greed and exploitation. Given the way they value human connection over cash, it's no surprise that many intelligent, competent Feelers (especially women) end up working in lower-paying, service-oriented jobs. Conversely, Feelers who are relatively well off may seek employment for altruistic, nonfinancial reasons—such as a desire to contribute to a particular organization with ideals and goals that resonate with their own.

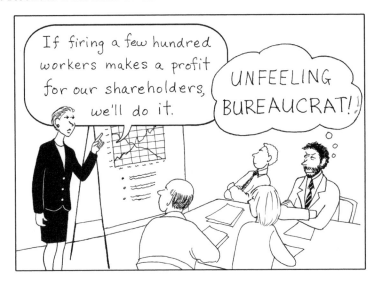

Feelers can do an excellent job at leading—if given the chance. But unfortunately, in many organizations the feeling preference is not valued.

Famous Feelers

Jimmy Carter, Princess Diana, Oprah Winfrey, Michael Jackson, Barbara Walters, Marie Osmond, Eleanor Roosevelt, Martin Luther King Jr., Joel Osteen, Magic Johnson, Elizabeth Taylor, Tammy Faye Bakker

It is only with the heart that one can see rightly;
what is essential is invisible to the eye.

ANTOINE DE SAINT-EXUPÉRY, *THE LITTLE PRINCE*

> Our feelings are our most genuine
> paths to knowledge.
>
> AUDRE LORDE

Male Feelers

In some ways, female Feelers are dealt a better hand in life than their male counterparts. Almost universally, women are socialized to be nurturing, sensitive, emotional, sympathetic, and compassionate—the very same traits, as it happens, that characterize the Feeling preference. Men who have a preference for feeling, however, often find themselves at odds with cultural expectations for males. As they grow up, they are chided for being too softhearted, emotional, "wimpy," or even unmasculine. Over and over, they receive the message (sometimes subtle, sometimes overt) that "real" men are rational, objective, tough-minded, independent, and unemotional. In other words, "real" men are Thinkers.

Boys with the Feeler preference learn at an early age that others—especially other men, sometimes even including their fathers—don't value their gentleness and compassion. To survive emotionally, such boys learn to judge and inhibit their feelings and continue to repress Feeler traits throughout their lives. In an attempt to prove their manhood, they may compensate by developing their rational side to the greatest extent possible or by presenting a cool, detached face to the world, or even by behaving in a sexually seductive manner. Despite such adaptations, however, the man with a Feeler preference remains inwardly sensitive, vulnerable, and desirous of the approval of others, although these traits may not be obvious to those who do not know him well.

On the other hand, there are some very positive aspects to being a Feeler male. For one thing, men with this personality preference usually relate well to women (better, in fact, than to other men). Ironically, Feeler men sometimes do better at establishing satisfying heterosexual relationships than do more "masculine" men. Feeler males also make inspiring leaders in conflict situations because of their unique blend of qualities—they convey a balance between strength and assertiveness, on the one hand, and concern and sympathy for others, on the other.

What Drives a Feeler Crazy

- People who are sparse with praise yet quick to point out problems

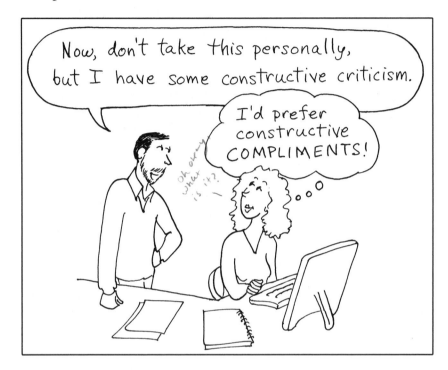

- People who worship logic and reason and therefore look for flaws in other people's thinking

---

Reason, with most people, means their own opinions.

WILLIAM HAZLITT

- Failing to take other people's feelings and concerns into consideration when making decisions

- Emotional unresponsiveness

> It is the devastating matter-of-factness which kills all romance.
>
> ELINOR GLYN

- Feeling undervalued, unappreciated, or taken for granted

- Being told—once again—that they're overly sensitive or too emotional

> Why is it that people who cannot show feelings presume that that is a strength and not a weakness?
>
> MAY SARTON

- Arguing just for sport

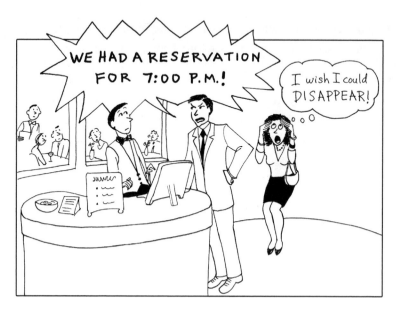

- Sarcasm, ridicule, put-downs

I'm a Feeler. Now What?

- Talk to yourself in nurturing, caring ways. Be as gentle with yourself as you are with others. Telling yourself things like "It'll be okay" (instead of "Oh, my God, this is terrible") or "Oops, let's try that one again" (instead of "Geez, I am such a loser") can make a big difference in your outlook.

- Search for employment that is consistent with your personal values. Avoid work environments where your warm and sensitive nature will not be appreciated.

- Practice observing your reactions to other people's remarks. See if you can simply name what you are feeling without getting caught up emotionally. Avoid personalizing statements that were not intended to be personal.

- Accept both sides of your nature, your anger as well as your benevolent feelings. Emotions aren't right or wrong—they just *are*.

- Tease out your own needs and inner thoughts, the ones that belong solely to you, not to your friends and family.

- Set limits and act assertively regarding issues that are important to you. Practice saying, "No," or, "Let me think about that," when others request your help. Then reflect on the effect that saying "Yes" would have on your schedule and your energy.

"No" uttered from the deepest
conviction is better and greater than a
"yes" merely uttered to please.

MAHATMA GANDHI

- Remember that conflict is not necessarily bad. An inevitable part of life, it can help you grow and change. The trick is not to avoid conflict but to learn from it.

- Ask for what you need. For extra credit, refrain from adding, "Is that *really* all right?" or, "Whatever you want is fine with me."

- Maintain healthy skepticism toward people in order to recognize those who don't have your best interests at heart. Get help in ending inappropriate relationships.

> Surround yourself with people who
> respect and treat you well.
>
> CLAUDIA BLACK

- Evaluate your own worth without depending on other people's views or opinions. Don't wait for someone else to tell you that you did well—go ahead and pat yourself on the back.

> Ultimately, love is self-approval.
>
> SONDRA RAY

8

The Thinker/Feeler
Relationship

In many areas of life—friendships and work relationships, for example—Thinkers and Feelers gravitate toward those who have the same preference. In intimate relationships, however, they often (and sometimes confusingly) find themselves drawn to each other.

A Thinker is often attracted to a Feeler's warmth and caring, as well as to his or her compassionate and nurturing ways. A Feeler can gently encourage a Thinker to be more understanding and sensitive and make it feel more comfortable for the Thinker to voice his or her frustrations, fears, and worries. For those who tend to keep their emotions to themselves, the opportunity to express them, while sometimes unnerving, can also be quite a relief.

The Feeler, on the other hand, can find the Thinker's rational or analytical style attractive, as well as the Thinker's ability to remain levelheaded in hard times and crises. Through modeling and encouragement, a Thinker can help a Feeler to be more objective and to react more positively to constructive criticism. A Thinker can also encourage an overly accommodating Feeler to stand up for himself or herself and avoid being taken advantage of.

In the beginning of a Thinker/Feeler relationship, both parties may be on their best behavior, each trying to please (or avoid displeasing) the other. Often, the Thinker will make an attempt to listen to the Feeler's feelings. The Feeler, in turn, will often make an effort to hold back expressions of strong emotions. But in time, their natural preferences inevitably reassert themselves, and the real relationship challenges are revealed.

Since the differences in behavior between a Thinker and a Feeler tend to be very obvious, both parties can frequently experience frustration and annoyance, and communication clashes can be intense. In many cases, the most significant problem has to do with expressions of appreciation. Feelers naturally communicate their deep emotions toward others and are lavish with expressions of love. Thinkers, by contrast, do not place as much value on intimacy as Feelers do and are not inclined to provide assurances of love and caring. In fact, their "personal" remarks to loved ones tend to focus, not on what they value, but on what they find fault with. In Thinker/Feeler relationships, then, Feelers are not only disappointed when Thinkers don't respond in kind to their warm sentiments, but hurt when they receive criticism instead of the kind of support they themselves offer so generously. Thinkers, conversely, are irritated by Feelers' predilection for over-the-top expressions of emotion and may perceive them as blatant exaggerations. Thinkers can also be genuinely puzzled by Feelers' sensitivity to criticism, perceiving it as a distressingly illogical reaction.

Conflict also typically arises between a Thinker and a Feeler around the issue of how they discuss each other's problems. Thinkers (especially, although not exclusively, male Thinkers) often rush to offer advice about how their partner should deal with any given difficulty and to suggest logical solutions. Then, having "fixed" the problem, they feel hurt when their partner ignores their advice and maybe even withdraws in annoyance. It can take a long time for a Thinker to understand that most people, especially Feelers, often just want to talk things through and know that they have been heard.

Though change is certainly possible for both parties in a Thinker/Feeler relationship, it can't be imposed from the outside. Attempts to coerce a Feeler partner into behaving more like a Thinker almost always backfire, as do the efforts of a Feeler to get a Thinker to express more understanding and compassion. Nonetheless, both Thinkers and Feelers often contribute to an "it's all your fault" dynamic, especially when each partner has a strong preference on the Thinker-Feeler scale.

Couples with more moderate preferences will often find it easier to compromise around their differing needs.

A relationship between two Thinkers doesn't present as many overt challenges as a Feeler/Thinker pairing. Both parties take pleasure in sharing different, even contradictory points of view, and they bring well-considered opinions to any discussion. They can engage in passionate intellectual debates without getting their feelings hurt. And when conflicts do arise, two Thinkers will analyze them logically, objectively, and impersonally. It can be hard, however, for either party to admit being wrong. They may not be especially romantic or sentimental, which suits them both—they don't need a lot of reassurance that they are loved, and they may even distrust the sentimentality. On the other hand, it may turn out that neither Thinker is really there for the other, especially when both are deeply absorbed in their own cognitive worlds. And even if both members of the couple want children, it may be that neither is willing to put a career on the back burner in order to raise a family.

A relationship between two Feelers has the potential to be warm and loving. Rather than thinking of their union as a practical alliance, Feelers often perceive themselves as having found a soulmate, especially when they share other preferences. Both sincerely want to support, please, and help the other. And because they share a deep desire to connect and share their innermost feelings, they're usually on the same page in terms of emotional bonding. On the downside, in their mutual desire for harmony, the Feeler couple can be overly cautious about avoiding conflict. If both of them tiptoe around problems that really need to be addressed, the relationship may eventually be threatened.

Neither a couple composed of two Feelers nor a couple composed of two Thinkers faces the same level of challenges that the Feeler/Thinker pair does. But even a strong Feeler and a strong Thinker, if they are capable of moving closer to the center of the continuum on occasion (usually those who are consciously working to develop greater balance), may find that their relationship improves accordingly. As always, it's important that each partner keep in mind that thinking and feeling are natural preferences. Like height or eye color, such preferences are not traits we purposely acquire to drive each other crazy.

But, whereas we can't really make ourselves taller or shorter or turn our brown eyes blue, we *can* learn more effective behaviors to make life—and love—a little easier.

Here are several techniques that I have found effective in improving communication, decreasing stress, and increasing respect between opposite-preference partners.

How to Get Along with a Thinker

- When you find that the wisdom, counsel, expertise, or advice of your Thinker partner is helpful, make sure you let him or her know. (A verbal thank-you is never out of line, and the occasional written note will be much appreciated, maybe even treasured.)

- Thinkers take constructive criticism as evidence that you have truly listened to them and understood their ideas. Engage with them on their level and offer feedback (critical or otherwise) that is accurate and precise.

- Let the Thinker in your life know that you appreciate his or her objectivity and ability to remain levelheaded and in control, especially in crisis situations.

- As a general rule, ask Thinkers what they *think* rather than how they *feel*. Sometimes a query about their emotional state may

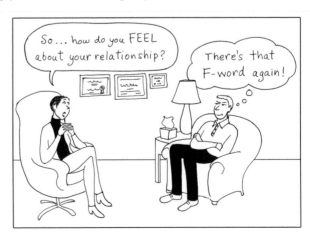

clearly be in order, but drop the subject if you meet resistance. Any pressure you apply is likely to backfire, causing the Thinker to become even more closed off.

- Avoid talking *excessively* about your feelings. If you need to tell your Thinker partner that he or she has offended or hurt you, wait until you have cooled down enough to communicate calmly and concisely. Otherwise, your words are apt to fall on deaf ears.

The sign of intelligent people is their ability to control emotions by the application of reason.

MARYA MANNES

- Make a point of engaging your Thinker partner in intellectually stimulating conversations. Every now and then, pretend that you're on the high school debate team and argue about an issue just for the fun of it. Not only do Thinkers enjoy this sort of exchange, but they respect those who can take a firm position and defend it.

- When your loved one offers constructive criticism, try to focus on the word "constructive." A Thinker's intentions are usually good, and he or she might even be surprised to know that others take such remarks personally.

- Don't sugarcoat your true thoughts. Be courteous and calm (if possible) when you express disagreement or dissatisfaction, but don't worry that hearing an unpleasant fact will hurt your partner's feelings in the same way that it might hurt yours. Vague or placating statements are more apt to irritate the Thinker than hard truths.

- Don't assume that your Thinker partner is unfeeling simply because he or she doesn't feel as you do.

- Remember that a Thinker can love deeply without ever mentioning the fact. You're not likely to receive frequent assurances of devotion, but that doesn't mean your partner *isn't* devoted. Notice all the nonverbal ways he or she expresses affection for you—and rent a romantic movie when you want to hear flowery speeches.

- Keep in mind that staying focused on tasks and projects is natural for a Thinker, not a rejection of your relationship.

Statements That Thinkers Hate to Hear

"You're so critical."
"You're heartless."
"You don't care about anyone but yourself."
"I asked how you feel, *not* what you think."
"You're thick-skinned."
"That hurts my feelings."

How to Get Along with a Feeler

I can live for two months on
a good compliment.

MARK TWAIN

- Be generous with personal expressions that show you care: these are nearly as vital to the Feeler's sense of well-being as food and water. Say "I love you" often, and don't stint on the hugs. Offer small, thoughtful expressions of affection (cards, e-mails, and "just because" gifts). To Feelers, the obvious doesn't speak for itself—they have to hear it and *feel* it.

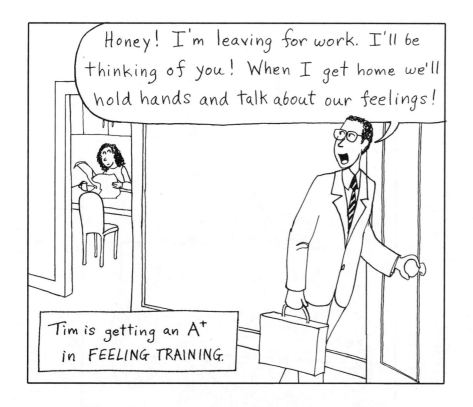

Tim is getting an A⁺ in FEELING TRAINING.

- Remember special occasions—anniversaries, birthdays, Mother's Day or Father's Day, and so on. Feelers assign great meaning to such remembrances, and if you happen to slip up and forget an important date, they can feel devastated and rejected.

- Respond, whenever you can comfortably do so, to your Feeler partner's desire for quality time with you. Try to cue in to signals that indicate a need for closer emotional connection. It may seem illogical, but if your partner has to ask for what he or she wants, getting it is not as satisfying.

- When your Feeler partner tells you how he or she is feeling, just listen. Let your partner talk things through without interrupting. A sympathetic expression is all that's really required of you here—don't try to solve the problem unless specifically requested to do so.

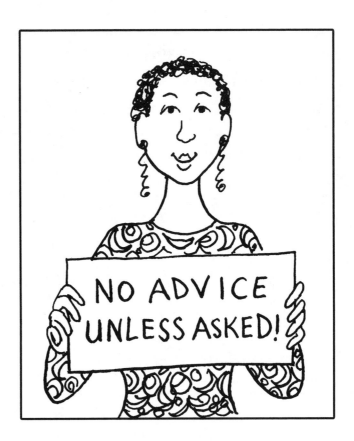

- No matter how well-meaning, your unsolicited criticisms will not be received as thoughtful gifts by your Feeler partner. You may be absolutely right about all the ways in which there is room for improvement. But for a warmer, friendlier relationship, it's best to keep most of your ideas about how your partner could change his or her behavior, appearance, worldview, and so on, to yourself.

Listening is a form of accepting.

STELLA TERRILL MANN

- Compliment your Feeler partner on what he or she does to make your relationship and home harmonious. If you don't tend to pick up on that sort of thing, challenge yourself to notice one nice thing your partner does each day—such as making dinner, straightening up the living room, helping you with a problem with an employee, or just asking how your day has been.

- Don't try prematurely to calm a Feeler partner who's upset. Feelers are usually able to see things more objectively after they've experienced their emotions.

- Be tolerant of your partner's need to express emotions, even if you don't feel the same urge yourself. One of the most common arguments in this type of opposite-preference relationship arises when the Thinker dismisses the Feeler's emotions as insignificant or unimportant. Remember that your partner's feelings are valid (as are yours) even if they don't make "logical" sense.

◦ The heart has its reasons which reason does not understand.

PASCAL

- When giving feedback, be gentle and tactful. Mention points of agreement before bringing up areas where your viewpoints diverge. And think carefully about your timing.

- When criticized, Feelers can withdraw, become insecure, and lose confidence. To their mind, no amount of praise or positive feedback is sufficient to cancel out one iota of negative feedback. When you hurt your partner's feelings, apologize.

- Value Feelers for who they are more than for what they do.

- Take time to learn who and what matters to your partner. For some people, this is a natural part of a relationship, but for others it requires conscious effort. You can find out a lot (and feel closer to your partner) by asking questions that demonstrate a positive interest in his or her friends, family, personal history, and so on.

- Enjoy cuddling that doesn't necessarily lead to sex. For the Feeler, the emotional aspect of love is just as important as the stuff that happens between the sheets.

Statements That Feelers Hate to Hear

"You're not being logical."

"You need to be objective about this."

"Why are you so sensitive?"

"Don't take this personally, but . . ."

9

The Lifestyle Preference

JUDGERS/PERCEIVERS

Read the following statements and check the sentence that describes you best—A or B. To achieve the most accurate score, answer the statements according to what is true for you, not according to what you would like to be true or think ought to be true.

The Inventory

1. A ☐ I make to-do lists and actually *do* the things on them.
   B ☒ I make to-do lists when I absolutely have to, but even then I don't necessarily follow them.

2. A ☐ When there's something I need to do, I try to get it done as soon as possible.
   B ☒ When there's something I need to do, I tend to procrastinate and to do everything but that.

3. A ☒ If I'm going someplace, I want to plan ahead of time, and I prefer to have the schedule settled before I leave the house.
   B ☒ I prefer leaving plans open-ended and going with the flow.

4. A ☐ I need to keep my things organized and orderly or the chaos will drive me crazy.

   B ☒ I consider myself organized, but my external surroundings can look chaotic to others.

5. A ☐ It's hard for me to relax until I've finished everything I have to do.

   B ☒ I can kick back and take it easy even if work is still pending.

6. A ☐ It frustrates me when a firm plan is already agreed on and other people want to change it, especially at the last minute.

   B ☒ Last-minute changes in plans don't bother me at all; in fact, I often enjoy them.

7. A ☐ I like to plan ahead as much as possible.

   B ☒ I like to improvise and adapt as I go.

8. A ☐ I prefer finishing a project before starting another one.

   B ☒ I'll often start a new project before finishing the one I'm on.

9. A ☒ I'm able to stay very focused on what I need to do.

   B ☒ Instead of staying on track, I am easily distracted by activities that aren't really priorities.

10. A ☐ I like to decide things as quickly as possible. I feel much more relaxed after a decision is made.

    B ☒ I tend to postpone decision-making so I can keep my options open as long as possible.

Scoring

In the first blank space below, record how many times you chose A as the answer to one of these ten questions. In the second blank space below, record how many times you chose B.

Total

___1___ A Judger

___10___ B Perceiver

Judgers and Perceivers in a Nutshell

This set of opposite styles determines whether we prefer to live our everyday outer lives in a more structured way (judging) or in a more spontaneous and open-ended way (perceiving).

Judgers are people who seek closure and who prefer to have matters settled and resolved as quickly as possible. They do not necessarily enjoy making decisions, but they do feel more comfortable once a decision is made. At that point, the matter is finally out of the way and off their mind; then they can go on to the next thing. People who prefer judging over perceiving are not necessarily more "judgmental" or less "perceptive."

Perceivers like to gather a lot of information and consider the different possibilities before they make a decision. Making decisions too quickly can be stressful to a Perceiver because it closes down other possibilities and options. In the language of personality types, perceiving means "preferring to take in information"; it does not mean "perceptive" in the sense of having quick and accurate perceptions about people and events.

As with the other three sets of opposite styles, no one behaves entirely one way or the other. We all have aspects of judging and perceiving within us, but within our core we prefer one way over the other.

The judging and perceiving preferences are most pronounced when people are dealing with the *outer* world—that is, when they are working or handling other obligations. When alone and doing just as they please, they are much more likely to show traits and behaviors of their opposite preference.

Some Judgers may come across as very decisive, disciplined, and structured at work, yet in their personal lives they are more flexible and spontaneous and have a strong desire to keep free time as open as possible. They would prefer that their plans not go awry, but if last-minute changes occur, they don't get all bent out of shape about it.

For some Perceivers, the pull toward flexibility and open-endedness is extremely strong; their stress levels rise like mercury when they're forced to make decisions before they're ready. Others don't like to make a decision on the spot, but if necessary they will do so without undue stress and be done with it. Like Judgers, Perceivers may behave one way at work and another way at home; some are highly adaptable and flexible in their private lives, yet shift into a more structured mode on the job.

Judgers represent about 60 percent of the American population, and Perceivers about 40 percent. In the United States, there is a great deal of pressure on people to act like Judgers in two major arenas of life—in the workplace and at school. Both institutions require punctuality, following the rules, and meeting deadlines—all of which are judging processes. Because Perceivers have no choice but to live in a judging world, they often adapt to its orderly ways in order to succeed, most typically on the job. As a result, many Perceivers *appear* to prefer judging—especially in the work environment—even though judging is not their natural preference.

Elsewhere in the world, Perceivers experience less pressure to conform—in some Latin American and Caribbean cultures, in fact, a judging preference may be seen as rigid and uptight. So, while Judgers and Perceivers live everywhere in the world, the preferences are valued differently from place to place—something to remember when you're planning your next vacation or fantasizing about the perfect lifestyle.

In a relationship, the differences in the behaviors of partners with high scores on these opposite preferences can be extremely frustrating to both. The contrast can be a chronic source of irritation and conflict especially for couples who live together, because each person's habits make an immediate, daily impact on the other.

JUDGERS

You Might Be a Judger If . . .

- Your favorite Christmas gift was a label maker; you use it all the time.

- "Whatever you want is fine with me" is not part of your normal vocabulary.

- You want to know what you are going to be doing tonight, next weekend, and next month.

- Poet Robert Frost looked back on the "road not taken"; you keep moving forward on the road ahead.

- Your idea of a mess looks organized to other people.

- You neatly refold the newspaper before you put it in the recycle bin.

- You are uncomfortable if a discussion does not end with a yes or no or an action plan.

- No joke, you really *would* divorce a mate who consistently forgot to replace the toothpaste cap.

Judgers at Their Best	Judgers at Their Worst
Efficient	Uptight
Conscientious	Rigid
Dependable	Bossy
Decisive	Controlling
Committed	Closed-minded
Purposeful	Inflexible
Organized	Overly scheduled
Industrious	Obsessive

Judgers 101

More than the rest of us, Judgers are uncomfortable with uncertainty. In any situation where a decision is up in the air, the Judger is the one pushing for definite and unambiguous closure. Judgers prefer to have matters settled as quickly as possible, not necessarily because they relish making decisions, but because they feel considerably more comfortable once things are resolved. When the issue is out of the way and off their mind, they feel ready to focus on the next item of business. Judgers are not known for making tentative plans or leaving arrangements open to last-minute changes. When they agree to a plan, they have every intention of carrying it out. Commitments are just that . . . commitments. Being asked to renegotiate or cancel set plans, cope with unexpected contingencies, or take on something completely unexpected at the last minute is stressful, irritating, and frustrating to a Judger.

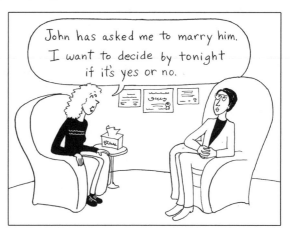

In their eagerness to wrap up the decision-making process, Judgers stop gathering information at a certain point and choose the best option available at the time. In so doing, they run the risk of making premature or inappropriate choices. Even when a decision has enormous consequences, they may rush through it, unable to tolerate extended uncertainty. And once they've settled on a course of action, they tend not to allow themselves to change their mind.

Organizing Style

> I gave my life to learning how to live.
> Now that I have organized it all . . .
> it's just about over.
>
> SANDRA HOCHMAN

Judgers thrive in an organized and orderly environment. Most find a cluttered space distracting and unsettling. Not all Judgers are immaculate housekeepers, but most feel more at ease when their things are where they belong. For Judgers, mess equals stress—whether it's their own or someone else's.

Loose ends and tasks left undone weigh on the Judger. That's why, in a Judger's home, dishes are usually washed and put away directly after a meal, files are kept in order, and paperwork is cleared off the desk as quickly as possible. Not only that, but bills are paid on time, and household finances adhere to a budget. A strong Judger has a system for organizing just about everything.

Time-out here for a moment. Of course, not every Judger in the world is a neat freak: for the sake of getting the basic idea across, I'm describing the most extreme end of the spectrum. Each preference on the Myers-Briggs Type Indicator scale, as I've said before, is expressed somewhere along a continuum from mild to extreme. But I'm sure if you or your partner is a Judger, you're feeling some familiarity here.

For Judgers who are also Intuitives, the well-organized area of their life is more likely to be their intellectual or creative world rather than their physical or tangible world. A writer or a professor, for example, might have very organized course chapter outlines and syllabi, yet leave dirty dishes drying out on the kitchen counter for days.

Judgers who are also Sensors are more likely to be organized about tangible things. These Judgers have clean closets, nicely detailed cars, and labeled hooks to hang their keys on.

When Judgers get up in the morning, they immediately want to know what the day is going to look like. "I'll just hang out and see how things develop" is not the Judger's style. Having routines and schedules provides a sense of security and comfort. Most Judgers make a daily to-do list, and crossing off items brings them a sense of completion. If a Judger happens to complete a task that's not on the list, he or she might even add it to the list retroactively—just for the satisfaction of crossing it off.

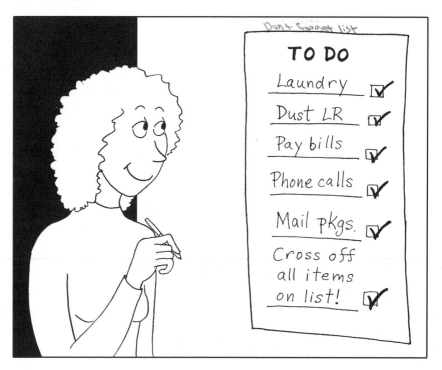

Take a look at a Judger's domestic life and you'll notice a strong sense of order and structure. Meals are planned beforehand (using shopping list, of course) and almost always served on time. Strong Judgers who are expecting guests for dinner may set the table the night before. Exercise routines are followed, gifts are purchased weeks or even months ahead of time, and all appropriate annual checkups for the entire family—including pets and vehicles—are put on the calendar. Some Judgers even schedule intimacy. A Judger leaves room for innovation and surprise, of course, but finds too much change without warning to be disconcerting.

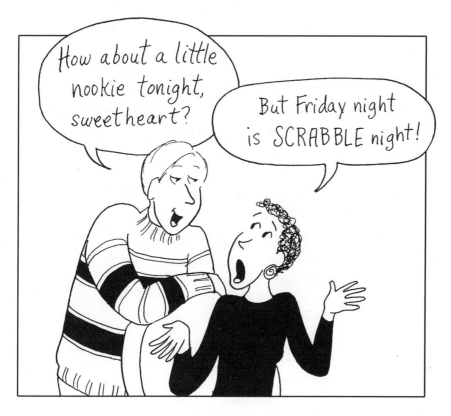

Time is of the essence to the busy Judger. Judgers are prompt, and they expect events to start on time. Having to wait for latecomers makes them irritable. When they're running the event themselves, they make sure that it begins promptly and adheres closely to the schedule.

When a vacation is coming up, strong Judgers will plan the itinerary and make reservations well in advance. They may allow some free time in the schedule, but not too much; they're concerned about making sure they accomplish all the things they intend to. However, to give themselves a break from their routines and schedules, some Judgers are more open-ended on vacations.

Conscientious and hardworking, Judgers put responsibilities before play. They'll make time to relax, but only after their work is done. But when, exactly, will that be? Because Judgers enjoy order and completion so much, they often have an endless number of things that need to be handled. Time for relaxing can be put off indefinitely as one to-do list flows right into the next. For those who are romantically involved with a Judger, it can be frustrating to always take a back seat to that never-ending agenda.

In the free time they allow themselves, Judgers often choose activities that provide them with a sense of purpose and accomplishment. A Judger might, for example, join the League of Women Voters or train for a half-marathon, as opposed to relaxing at the beach or lying back in their La-Z-Boy with a book. Judgers tend to find the retirement years rough going at first; all that unstructured time can be unsettling. In short order, however, most have dedicated themselves to a steady hobby or a project.

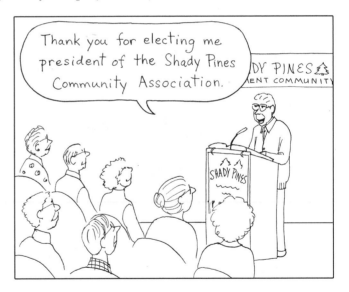

Communicating with a Judger

When Judgers speak out on an issue, you can tell where they stand. Unlike their Perceiver opposites, they are fond of declarative statements that end with an exclamation point. Their speech may be peppered with "shoulds" and "oughts" that not only apply to others but also to themselves. Strong Judgers often see things as right or wrong, good or bad, black or white. Their statements convey a sense of purpose and direction, and they rarely straddle the fence but come down firmly on one side or the other. All this tends to lend a parental or authoritarian quality to a Judger's definitive communication style. Intuitive Judgers (NJs) are more willing to explore thoughts, ideas, and feelings, but still have a need to come to some conclusion.

Judgers don't mind discussing general issues, but they prefer that people stay focused on the topic at hand and not wander off on tangents or side discussions. Too much talk slows progress and delays resolution. In their desire to bring a discussion to closure, they can come off sounding brisk, officious, or impatient, especially when they're also Thinkers (TJs).

Judgers at Work

In the American workplace, Judgers are held in high esteem. Within most organizations, the time management system favors the Judger's style. The reason is obvious: Judgers get results! Unlike their opposite type, Perceivers, they're not as interested in discussions that explore all the angles. And while Judgers may step on a few toes along the way, their willpower and sense of resolve often lead to impressive results.

When beginning a task or project, Judgers don't leave much to chance. Efficiently and thoroughly, they map out the necessary steps and know how things should work to get a system in place. Whether working alone or with others, they follow an outline and cover all the essential points.

Judgers tend to begin a task or assignment ahead of schedule to ensure that it will be finished when it's supposed to be. They plan the timeline accurately and meet the deadline reliably, often with time to spare. The last thing a Judger wants to do is wait until the last minute to finish up a project and experience the resulting internal anxiety. Judgers also can find it unsettling to juggle multiple projects; they often prefer to tackle just one job at a time so that they can move ahead with full focus on it until it's done.

You won't find a Judger who is reluctant to step up into a position of power, at least not an extraverted Judger. In any field, the Judger's decisive decision-making style lends itself to higher-level positions such as manager, supervisor, or administrator. Many prefer being in charge so that they can take control and provide direction—*their* direction. *After all,* the Judger thinks, *I know what needs to be done, and if I don't handle it, it will never get done. And even if it does get done, it won't be done right!* It may not surprise you to learn that most bosses are moderate to strong Judgers. Judgers tend to be more comfortable with authority, hierarchy, and rules than Perceivers.

Judgers excel in—and are most fulfilled by—careers that call upon their strengths in creating structure and organization. Since organizational skills are in fact the backbone of many careers, Judgers flourish in diverse situations.

Famous Judgers

Hillary Clinton, Dr. Laura, Judge Judy, Martin Luther King Jr., Billy Graham, Oprah Winfrey, Sam Donaldson, Maria Shriver, Ted Koppel, Bryant Gumbel, Arthur Ashe, Kristi Yamaguchi, Nancy Kerrigan, Peter Jennings

---

> Once a decision was made, I did not
> worry about it afterward.
>
> HARRY S TRUMAN

> A peacefulness follows any decision,
> even the wrong one.
>
> RITA MAE BROWN

What Drives a Judger Crazy

- People who can't commit to a definite plan

- People who wait until the last minute to make a decision

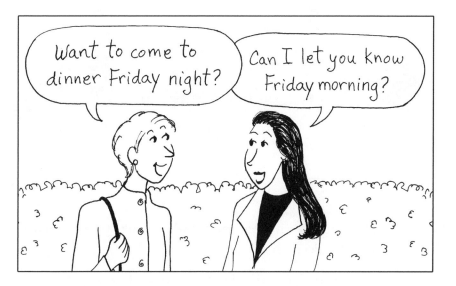

- Disorganization, mess, and clutter

- People who aren't punctual

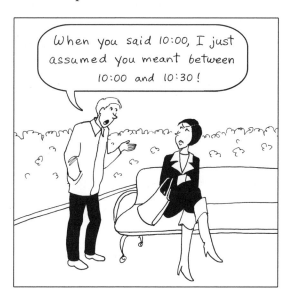

- Those who take forever to make even a simple decision

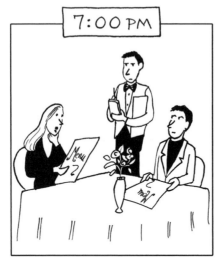 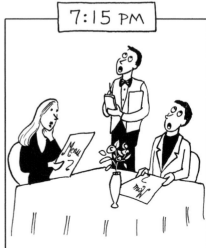

- Being presented with more options when you're trying to move ahead with a decision

- People who aren't realistic about how long a task will take to finish—so that you have to finish it for them!

There are two different kinds
of people in this world: those who
finish what they start, and.

BRAD RAMSEY

- An overdose of ambiguous statements such as:

    "I don't know."

    "It doesn't matter to me."

    "Anything you decide is okay with me."

    "Whatever."

I'm a Judger. Now What?

- Once in a while, focus on what you *want* to do rather than on what you *should* do. For one week, try "giving" yourself an hour each day to do whatever you happen to feel like doing at that moment—no preplanning allowed. Notice how that freedom feels (sensational? scary? somewhere in between?) and which activities truly give you pleasure.

- Learn to go with the flow and enjoy the moment for what it is.

> Slow down and enjoy life. It's not
> only the scenery you miss by going too fast—
> you also miss the sense of where
> you are going and why.
>
> EDDIE CANTOR

- Keep in mind that life is not a to-do list.

- When making important decisions about your life, take the time to explore different options. Don't be in a rush, especially with choices that may have major or long-term repercussions, either for you or for others.

- Practice leaving your choices open some of the time. And remember, it's not illegal to change your mind.

- Be sure to apply your need for closure to yourself, not to others!

- Instead of automatically giving answers or offering advice, ask questions and listen to the input and opinions of other people.

- Remember that others may not share your need for structure and order. As much as you want them to conform to your ways, be willing to try some of their ways too (even if, deep down, you are pretty sure their way is not even in the same ballpark as yours).

- When you see that someone didn't clean up after themselves or completely ignored your instructions—*breathe*. Realize that *you* may have to do many of the things you really want done yourself—all by yourself.

- Have your own room—or your own house!

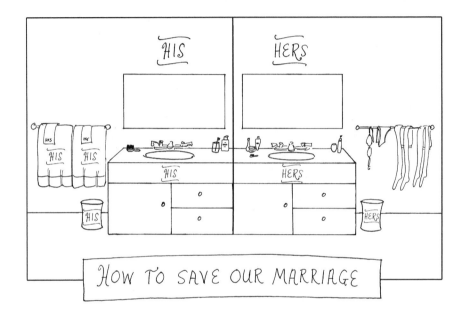

There is much to be done; therefore
we must proceed slowly.

BUDDHA

PERCEIVERS

You Might Be a Perceiver If . . .

√ • When going on a weekend car trip, you like to just take off, trusting that you'll enjoy the adventure as you go.

• On most mornings, you spend ten minutes looking for your keys or cell phone or both.

√ • When doing the dishes, you are likely to leave a pan or two in the sink but still consider the job done.

• You once looked for your MasterCard statement in the "M" section of your file cabinet . . . and there it was!

• You can spend days, even months, collecting data before purchasing an item.

• You got through college by pulling all-nighters.

• The toll booth operator always looks a little disapproving when you hand over your crumpled bills.

• You are a piler, not a filer.

• You've run out of gas more than once; maybe you've even had your electricity turned off because you forgot to pay the bill.

Perceivers at Their Best	Perceivers at Their Worst
Flexible ✓	Noncommittal
Adaptable ✓	Unreliable
Curious ✓	Flaky
Easygoing ✓	Disorganized
Open-minded ✓	Forgetful ✓
Nonjudgmental ✓	Unfocused ✓
Spontaneous ✓	Undisciplined
Casual ✓	Unpredictable

Perceivers 101

*Some persons are very decisive when
it comes to avoiding decisions.*

BRENDAN FRANCIS

It is easier for Perceivers to determine what they *don't* want rather than what they do want. When it's time to make a final decision, they

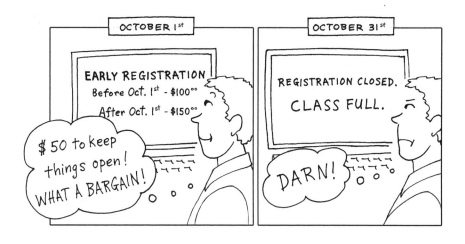

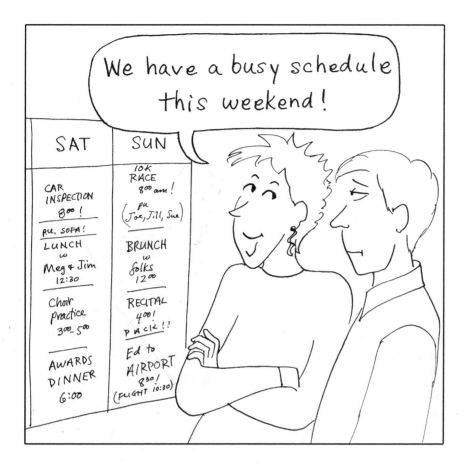

tend to procrastinate—what if something better shows up? It might, of course. On the other hand, Perceivers often miss out on events and experiences because they let crucial deadlines pass.

Before making a decision, Perceivers gather information for as long as possible and consider a wide variety of alternatives and possibilities. Settling on a plan too quickly is unappealing to them because other, potentially more interesting or exciting possibilities might present themselves. With all the options out there, Perceivers have a hard time narrowing their focus and discerning what is most important. Sometimes their indecisiveness overwhelms them. (It certainly can overwhelm others!) But they resent pressure to make a definite plan or commitment.

> Often greater risk is involved in postponement
> than in making a wrong decision.
>
> HARRY A. HOPF

Organizing Style

Perceivers prefer to live in a spontaneous, open-ended way, letting life unfold as it may. They prefer a lifestyle that allows them to be responsive to the needs and desires of the moment. Perceivers don't mind improvising and adapting to changes in plans. Many even enjoy the unexpected. This doesn't mean that they like being startled or surprised, but that they are comfortable with minimal planning and predetermination.

Perceivers don't like feeling hemmed in, obligated, or restricted. They keep weekends and days off as open as possible so they can do what they want, when they want. This is not to say that Perceivers never make any plans whatsoever—often they have a general idea of what they intend to do, but it's always open to change. They often throw a meal together spontaneously and do chores and exercise when the mood strikes. Socializing tends to be spur of the moment too—at least if the Perceiver has anything to say about it.

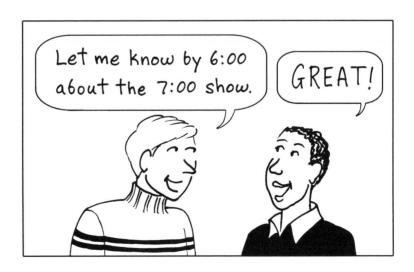

Perceivers enjoy variety and dislike being tied to just one way of doing things. Often a Perceiver undertakes a chore or task (preparing a dinner for guests, redecorating a room, planning a trip) with one idea in mind, then makes adjustments as newer, more intriguing ideas present themselves.

> I am one of those who never knows the direction
> of my journey until I have almost arrived.
>
> ANNA LOUISE STRONG

A Perceiver's style is to go back and forth between one task and another. Right in the middle of one project, they'll often start a second and maybe go on to a third as well. This way of operating may appear chaotic, but it makes perfect sense to the Perceiver. And should an impulse to relax suddenly strike, it doesn't bother the Perceiver to leave something (or everything, for that matter!) incomplete.

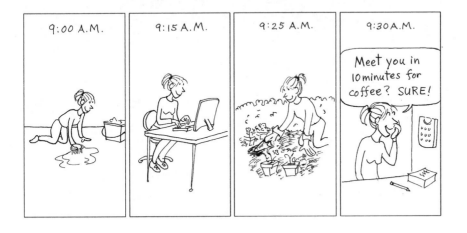

It is quite possible for Perceivers to be efficient at organizing belongings that matter to them, especially those associated with work, hobbies, or personal projects. In areas that are less interesting to a Perceiver, however, disorganization is likely to reign. Frequently used items are usually just left out in the open rather than put away. Some

Perceivers do prefer a neat home or workspace, but have a relaxed attitude about making sure it stays that way. Fortunately for them, Perceivers are perfectly able to function in the middle of what others would consider disarray.

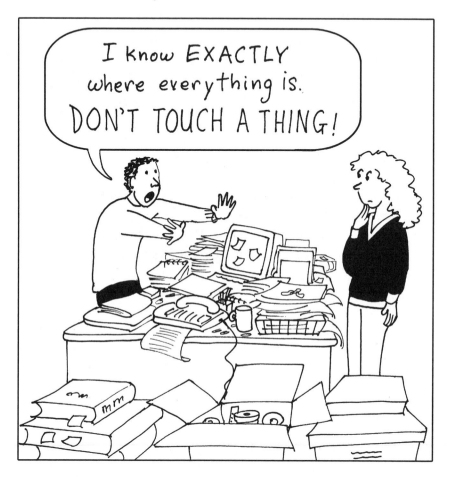

Don't get the wrong idea: Perceivers recognize the need for organization. They may even be in the habit of making to-do lists, although they're not particularly adept at following them. In fact, a Perceiver may not remember to look at the list once it's been created and may even lose it.

Despite an underlying suspicion that lists and other organizational tools stifle spontaneity and creativity, Perceivers sometimes go to great lengths to become more organized, developing elaborate systems to keep themselves on track. But creating a new system is often more satisfying than actually using it. Once the novelty wears off, Perceivers tend to revert to their old ways . . . until the next time around.

I write down everything I want to remember.
That way, instead of spending a lot of
time trying to remember what it is
I wrote down, I spend the time looking
for the paper I wrote it down on.

ANONYMOUS

Getting a handle on personal finances can be quite challenging for some Perceivers. Bills may be paid late, checkbooks left unbalanced, budgets created and then forgotten. Strong Perceivers are especially prone to allowing tasks they see as tedious to take a back seat to everything else.

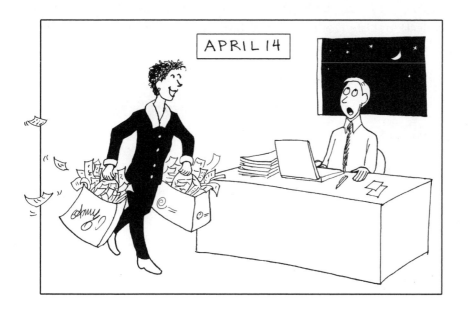

Communicating with a Perceiver

Sometimes it's hard to gauge a Perceiver's views or opinions for one simple reason: they themselves may not know what they are. Open-minded and curious, Perceivers are able to see issues from all sides. The opinion of each new person they talk to and each additional article or book they read makes an impression and has an impact. On the positive side, people are drawn to Perceivers because they take others' ideas seriously. On the other hand, it can be frustrating for all involved when the Perceiver simply cannot land firmly on one side of an issue or the other.

Perceivers approach discussion as an exploratory mission. They often ask questions to stimulate ideas and to seek alternative ways of looking at issues, not to solicit definitive answers. The right choice, they trust, will somehow emerge from the discussion. Perceivers are oriented toward possibilities, and a satisfying discussion or debate includes plenty of time for tangents and side discussions. Unlike the Judger, who tends to dispense with issues a bit too hastily, the Perceiver never quite wants to let go and will press to revisit a done deal if new insights or information surface.

You can often identify the Perceiver in the crowd simply by vocal inflection. Listen for statements that end with question marks instead of periods and sentences that trail off:

"So far as I know . . ."

"Maybe . . . but I'm not sure. I could be wrong."

"Whatever . . ."

"It could be . . ."

Perceivers at Work

Perceivers seek a work environment that allows for variety and change. If at all possible, they enjoy a flexible and varied work schedule, such as working from 7:00 A.M. to 3:00 P.M. at the office one day, then working from home the next. Perceivers are inclined to question and rebel against authority and rules that restrict their freedom and spontaneity.

Perceivers like to start new projects, but completing them is a different matter. Even after a project is well under way, it's difficult for Perceivers to shut down their receptivity to new ideas. The tendency is to keep gathering information—much more, in fact, than may be needed. This continuous influx of new data demands the constant reworking of decisions and plans. Consequently, the Perceiver's ideas may not be translated into action in a timely fashion, and sometimes the original plan is never even carried out.

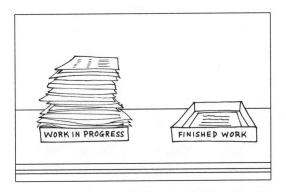

WORK IN PROGRESS   FINISHED WORK

Time slips away from Perceivers easily, especially when they're working for themselves and don't report to anyone. To meet the deadlines that always seem to descend upon them too soon, Perceivers resort to last-minute spurts of energy. As the deadline closes in, they can feel frazzled and frantic. But when they're under a real time crunch and must deliver, the adrenaline kicks in and they work more efficiently. Too many deadlines, however, feel constraining and confining, and they may rebel against the pressure. For obvious reasons, Perceivers prefer deadlines that are more flexible and open to negotiation. The job will get done . . . eventually.

> I love deadlines. I like the whooshing
> sound they make as they fly by.
>
> DOUGLAS ADAMS

Most conventional workplaces favor a Judger's more fastidious and efficient approach. The Perceiver's tendency toward nontraditional attitudes (and, sometimes, behavior) doesn't always go over well in a highly structured environment. Rather than take responsibility when something goes wrong, Perceivers like to cut themselves some slack. Add to the mix a chronic reluctance to make decisions and a relaxed attitude toward deadlines and you can see why a typical Perceiver might not be named Businessperson of the Year. Nonetheless, Perceivers often possess striking leadership qualities, chief among them curiosity, open-mindedness to new ideas, and genuine interest in what others have to offer. In times of flux and uncertainty, the flexible Perceiver remains a model of cool serenity. And when being organized is absolutely necessary, a Perceiver can sometimes even access his or her opposite-side preference and temporarily function like a Judger.

Famous Perceivers

Cloris Leachman, Andy Rooney, Johnny Cash, Lucille Ball, Eddie Murphy, Goldie Hawn, James Taylor, Martin Short, Tom Cruise, Clint Eastwood, Patrick Swayze, Marilyn Monroe, Magic Johnson, Paul McCartney

If your house is really a mess and a stranger comes to the door, greet him with, "Who could have done this? We have no enemies."

PHYLLIS DILLER

What Drives a Perceiver Crazy

- People who close off discussions too quickly because they're so eager to settle matters

- People who think that they have made a definite commitment to a plan when, in fact, it was merely up for consideration

---

One possible reason why things aren't going
according to plan is that there never was a plan.

ASHLEIGH BRILLIANT

- People who believe that a right way ~~really~~ *is perfect* exists

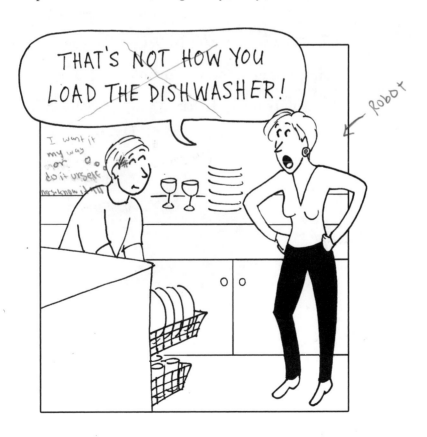

- People who get an ulcer when someone is running a few
  minutes late

I have noticed that the people
who are late are often so much
jollier than the people who have
to wait for them.

E. V. LUCAS

- Being forced to make a hasty decision

- Invitations for events far in the future

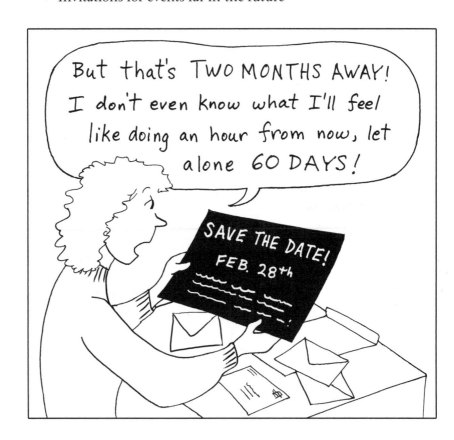

I'm a Perceiver. Now What?

- Make sure you allow yourself the flexibility and spontaneity that you crave in your free time. If you can't manage it any other way, play hooky or take a "mental health day" every once in a while.

- Each day make a short list of tasks that need to be completed. (That's "short" as in "not long.") Focus on only one task.

- Break large jobs down into manageable pieces. Acknowledge your progress, possibly with a small reward—or possibly just by saying, "Good job, me!"—when you meet each goal.

- Starting right now, stop automatically saying yes to new projects. Take out your calendar, put on your thinking cap, and seriously consider whether you can squeeze in one more activity or endeavor, given your existing obligations and time constraints.

- Don't force yourself to do a task the same old way. Follow your heart and try out the experimental method or technique that makes it beat a little faster.

- Consider taking a course in time management. It can be frustrating to deal with someone who is chronically late or who fails to follow through. Addressing the situation directly is an act of compassion for your friends, family, and co-workers— and in the long run, for yourself.

- Avoid spending too much time considering an endless list of possibilities. Learn when it's time to make a decision on the basis of the available information. As the saying goes, "Fish or cut bait."

- Make sure you have your own space, to keep however you like.

- Give others general rather than specific time frames regarding your plans. That way, you won't feel as oppressed by the clock, and they won't feel as frustrated with you.

- When someone pesters you to move more quickly, tell that person that nagging just makes you dig in your heels. What's more, it makes you horribly passive-aggressive.

I had a terrible fight with my wife on
New Year's Eve. She called me a
procrastinator. So I finished addressing
the Christmas cards and left.

ROBERT ORBEN

10

The Judger/Perceiver Relationship

As with all opposites, Judgers and Perceivers can find each other quite appealing as potential romantic partners. Each may sense that the other fills in some missing aspect of themselves, providing a welcome balance. And in the early stages of infatuation, tensions tend to resolve themselves quite nicely in the bedroom. But when a Judger and a Perceiver attempt to form a committed relationship, they often find the differences between their natural behaviors to be extremely challenging. In fact, the Perceiver may develop what amounts to a love-hate relationship with the Judger, while the Judger, similarly, continues to find the Perceiver attractive, but also chronically annoying. In the beginning of a relationship, both parties are apt to be on their best behavior. The Judger may attempt to be more receptive and adaptable, while the Perceiver often makes an effort to be more orderly and decisive. But in time, their natural preferences reassert themselves.

Most conflicts in a Judger/Perceiver relationship stem from the discrepancy between the Judger's need for order and structure and the Perceiver's need for flexibility and open-endedness. The Judger becomes stressed by the Perceiver's ever-changing plans and seemingly lax approach to accomplishing tasks—or often enough, *not* accomplishing them. By the same token, the Perceiver finds the Judger's ideas about the right and wrong ways of doing things oppressive and even demoralizing. Eventually, opposite-preference partners will attempt to coerce each other into more compatible behavior. But imposing restrictive time frames on a Perceiver, or pressuring him or her to commit to plans, usually ends in resentment. And the Perceiver who tries to get the Judger to loosen up and go with the flow will likewise encounter resistance. Without outside help, or learning about preferences, the couple may end up in continual conflict, extinguishing the romantic spark initially ignited by their differences. This dysfunctional dynamic is especially common when each partner has a strong preference on the judging-perceiving scale. Couples with more moderate preferences usually find it easier to compromise around their differing needs.

Partners who share a preference for either judging or perceiving have a much easier time in some ways, although the alignment of their other three preferences also, of course, affects their overall compatibility. In a relationship between two Judgers, both usually feel supported in their need to complete tasks promptly, to make plans well in advance, and to avoid abrupt changes of all kinds. The tendency they share to value the security and stability of a committed relationship makes them especially motivated to work out any problems that arise. But on the downside, two Judgers can be quite inflexible about schedules and routines. They may also find themselves locked in a perpetual power struggle, both of them continually wrestling for control and insisting that their way—and *only* their way—is the right one.

Two Perceivers can get along well as long-term romantic partners. Each respects the other's need for freedom and spontaneity, for space and open-ended time. Both adapt to change with ease. Both make time to relax and have fun together, whether or not they've finished their work. But you can imagine the domestic chaos that results in the typical two-Perceiver couple as each procrastinates about chores, paperwork, and most other practical needs and obligations. If both are strong Perceivers, the level of disorder can become quite extreme.

To keep things running at least somewhat smoothly and efficiently, one of the pair usually ends up taking a quasi-Judger role. Someone, after all, has to load the dishwasher, fold the laundry, keep medical appointments, return phone calls, get the children off to school on time, and so on. Such tasks fall on the partner who has a stronger desire for neatness and more free time or, in many cases, on the woman. To the outside world, a Perceiver who assumes most of the household's responsibilities may look very much like a Judger. Inside, however, this partner usually resents having his or her freedom curtailed. For the relationship to succeed, these two Perceivers need to come up with fair and reasonable systems that enable them to handle mundane tasks while accommodating their natural way of being. (Hiring a housekeeper, for example, has rescued more than one Perceiver/Perceiver relationship from disaster.)

Once again, it's important to keep in mind that judging and perceiving are natural preferences, not behaviors that opposite-preference partners purposely adopt to drive each other crazy. Understanding makes us less judgmental about ways of being that differ from our own and leads us toward acceptance and appreciation. In fact, the obvious obstacles notwithstanding, a Judger/Perceiver relationship has much to offer those who are open to personal growth. Each partner can count on the other's strengths to compensate for and supplement his or her own weaknesses. And eventually they may even learn to embody the positive opposite qualities they see in each other. So when the Perceiver feels that familiar flare of annoyance at the Judger's orderliness, or when the Judger grows irate over the Perceiver's indifference to structure, both need to stop and reflect on the big picture. These differences, after all, were part of the initial attraction. And when two contrasting approaches to life are better understood within the context of a relationship, they can complement each other and bring balance instead of causing problems.

Here are several techniques that I have found to be effective in improving communication, decreasing stress, and increasing respect between opposite-preference partners.

How to Get Along with a Judger

- Be mindful of a Judger's desire for an orderly environment by remembering to pick up after yourself and put things where they belong. Keep common working or living areas free of clutter. Be sure to initiate and complete your share of household chores, regardless of whether you're a man or a woman.

- When you borrow something, be sure to return it, and in the condition in which it was lent to you.

- Pay more attention to time, especially when tardiness will affect your Judger partner. If you're running late, call.

- When you say you'll do something—picking up clothes at the cleaners or milk from the store, getting back to your partner with a phone number, finding a caterer for cousin Lizzie's graduation party—do it.

- If your Judger partner asks a yes-or-no question, give him or her a yes-or-no answer. Period.

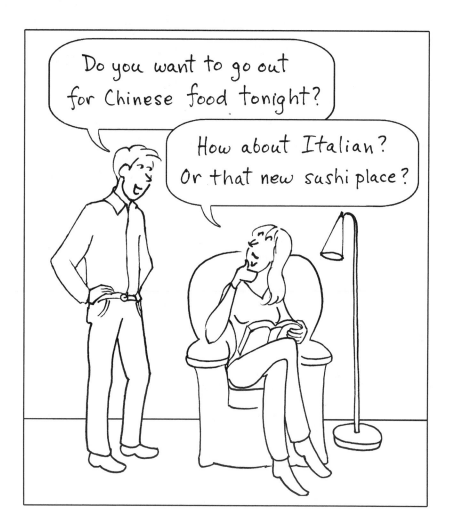

- Honor your agreements and commitments. Don't keep things up in the air too long. Avoid last-minute changes or cancellations whenever possible.

- When you want physical intimacy, let your partner know so that he or she can mentally prepare for it.

- Plan ahead so that you're prepared with thoughtful gifts and cards.

- Minimize interruptions and surprises. Don't spring things on your partner and expect a positive reaction.

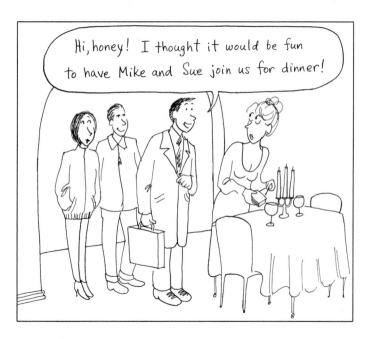

Statements That Judgers Hate to Hear

"Try to be more flexible."
You're uptight!"
"Loosen up."
"Stop stressing, it'll get done."
"You're being controlling."
"You always think you're right."

How to Get Along with a Perceiver

- Give your Perceiver partner a lot of freedom and latitude. Don't box in your partner with too many schedules or plans.

- Keep in mind that when pressured to meet a deadline, a Perceiver can become even more scattered or forgetful and run even later.

- When making a request or asking a Perceiver to do a task, leave that person room to do things his or her own way. Avoid nagging, especially about small annoyances or chores left undone. Trust that your partner will get things done, even if in a time frame that is different from yours.

- Let your Perceiver partner know when it's really important that he or she follow through with a plan or task; otherwise, try to be flexible.

- Give your Perceiver partner general rather than specific time frames.

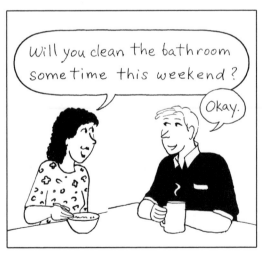 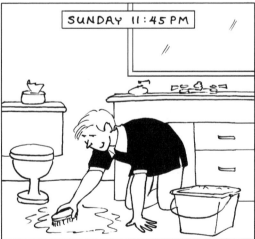

- Participate in some of the off-the-cuff activities your partner suggests.

- Be open to spontaneous lovemaking. Let your partner show you some unexpected pleasure and new experiences. Indulge his or her need to have sex at different times and in different places.

- Respect your partner's need to gather a lot of information before making a decision. Don't force a Perceiver to rule out options prematurely.

- When your partner thinks aloud about changes, avoid overreacting.

Statements That Perceivers Hate to Hear

"You've got your head in the clouds." ✓
"Can't you ever make up your mind?" ✓
"Just do it!" ✓
"Just decide!" ✓
"Pick a side!" ✓
"You sure start a lot of things, but . . ."
"You're being a flake."

11

Final Thoughts

---

*Find the person who will love you because
of your differences and not in spite of them
and you have found a lover for life.*

LEO BUSCAGLIA

Can This Relationship Work?

No relationship is perfect, and no one person is perfect for you. If you're waiting for the perfect person, you'll probably have to wait a long time. But with the knowledge about yourself and others that you've gained from reading this book and taking the inventories, you are in a much better position to enjoy and improve any relationship you are in.

In my many years as a therapist, I've noted that the most promising scenario for a relationship occurs when two people have some similar preferences that provide them with common ground and some differences that bring interest and balance to the relationship. Studies show that most couples have two or three preferences in common; very few couples have all four in common. The more preferences you have in common with your partner, the more likely it is that the two of you will understand and get along with each other and know how to meet each other's need for love. In every relationship, however, whether the partners are very similar, very different, or someplace in between, it's vital that they really "see" each other and stay open to learning about each other over time.

Having three or four sets of preferences in common does not guarantee a wonderful "happily ever after" relationship. It does not mean that you will always get along well or agree with each other. When the person you are with is similar to you, it can sometimes seem as though he or she is holding up a mirror to traits and behaviors you may dislike in yourself. Personal tendencies you may be blind to can become obvious when you see someone else acting as you do. While this type of revelation can lead to change and growth, it can also cause unhappiness and conflict.

In a relationship between two very similar individuals, it is often the case that one of them finds himself or herself automatically using the opposite preferences more to help them function better as a couple. In earlier chapters, I have pointed out the specific types of accommodations that the more flexible partner is likely to make. Sometimes this shift leads to chronic resentment on the part of the adaptive partner. When we have no choice but to deny our innate preferences, stress is almost always the result. It's interesting to note, however, that Jung believed that people find it easier to sustain a satisfying relationship with a similar-preference partner in the second half of life. By then, we are likely to have developed our opposite preferences and be capable of using whatever mode we need in a given situation without too much stress.

Although having fewer preferences in common can spell more difficulty for a couple—and consequently, more need for adjustment— great relationships can happen between people regardless of how many preferences they share. The less similar you are to your partner, however, the greater the likelihood of miscommunication and misunderstanding.

The success of any relationship is based on the ability to negotiate and compromise—not on what happens in the bedroom, despite the impression conveyed by popular culture. When we are able to acknowledge, respect, and work with our differences, an opposite-preference relationship can be deeply loving and satisfying. And as I have noted throughout this book, differences are not merely unfortunate obstacles to overcome; they can enrich our lives and help us grow by exposing us to the less developed parts of our own personality.

In any relationship, those with one or more particularly strong preferences need to make sure that they don't try to force their ways on their partner. When you think that your way is the only "right" one, your relationship is bound to suffer. The fact is that you can never really change someone else. When you try, your partner only feels misunderstood, controlled, and resentful. And imagine that you *did* somehow accomplish this feat—you'd probably no longer find your partner nearly as interesting.

> Why does a woman work ten years to
> change a man's habits and then complain
> that he's not the man she married.
>
> BARBRA STREISAND

As you gain an understanding of personality preferences, you can more easily see things from your partner's perspective. It's important to use your knowledge of the Myers-Briggs system for the good of the relationship and not as justification for your own behaviors. Neither you nor your partner should consider a preference an excuse to be insensitive.

It's also important not to take advantage of your knowledge of personality typing to label your partner, especially in a noncomplimentary way. Labeling is the downside of understanding personality preferences. Isabel Myers refused to tolerate negative labeling. I once read that when a student used a derogatory adjective to describe a personality preference, she would gently substitute another adjective with the same intent—but in a more neutral tone. "You mentioned 'pigheaded,'" she'd say. "Did you mean 'firm'?"

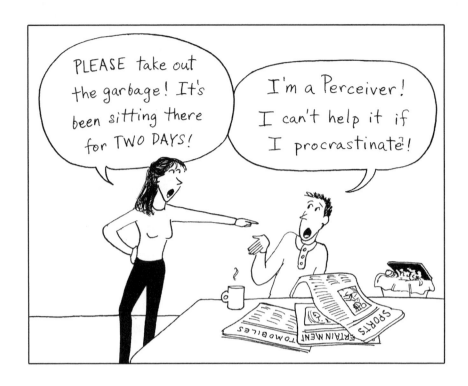

Try to avoid paying too much attention to the ways in which you and your partner are not ideally suited. Instead, focus on what you enjoy doing as a couple, whether that's quietly coexisting in the same space, traveling to exotic lands, throwing dinner parties for your friends, watching bad TV in your sweats, or slipping between the sheets.

Finally, I hope you are now in a better position to have a few good laughs about yourself and to take a lighter and more humorous look at your weaknesses and foibles and those of others.

Even though you've nearly reached the end of this book, I hope you'll continue to investigate the intriguing realm of personality preferences long after you turn the final page. To learn more about your four-letter MBTI type, see Appendix A. To make the most of what you have discovered in reading these chapters, you will need to use this new knowledge on a regular basis or you will forget it.

Here are some partner exercises to reinforce your awareness of personality preferences and enhance your relationship in general.

Exercise 1: Dialogue

Although you probably have a good idea about your partner's preferences on a few dimensions, ask your partner to read the book or do the inventories, look at the "How to Get Along with . . ." sections, and check the items that apply to him or her. Do the same yourself. Have a dialogue about one of the points raised by this exercise. One at a time, have a dialogue about all of the different points it brings up.

Changing one annoying behavior in one preference area can have a positive impact on your relationship as a whole. For instance, giving your introverted partner more time alone or not pressuring a Thinker to talk about his or her feelings may lead to surprising openings that have never before been experienced in the relationship.

Exercise 2: Write-Read-Share

Take some time to write the answers to the following questions. Suggest that your partner do the same. Then take turns reading what each of you has written.

What do you like best about your relationship?

What makes you feel happy and loved?

What makes you feel closer to your partner?

What pushes you apart?

How does your partner show appreciation for you?

What does your partner do that annoys you?

Exercise 3: Mutual Appreciation

Each day, take five minutes to share what you appreciate about your partner. Then share two things that *you* (not your partner) could have done differently to make the relationship better. For instance, "I could have reacted less angrily when you asked me to go to your parents'. And I wish I had woken you up with a kiss instead of letting the alarm clock do the job."

As I said in the beginning, the study of personality preferences has been an important part of my life for many decades. I am glad to have shared this valuable information with you and hope that learning about personality preferences has deepened your self-understanding and will help you honor and develop the strengths and abilities you bring to your relationships. Even now, forty years after I first began to study the MBTI preferences, I continue to gain new and useful insights that help me in all my relationships, whether with friends, colleagues, or family members. May your own investigations prove to be similarly rich and rewarding.

It is not our purpose to become each other;
it is to recognize each other, to learn to see
the other and honor him for what he is.

HERMANN HESSE

Where Do You Go from Here?

Although I'd written five books about personality type—including one that helps couples have the most satisfying relationships—I was having trouble helping two friends who were struggling in their relationship understand how it was really their *type* differences that were getting in their way.

Not surprising, one was very Extraverted, and the other quite Introverted. At about the same time, I received a review copy of this book. Intrigued by the title, and a fan of Renee, I dove in. Beginning with the first page, I experienced Renee's gift for explaining type preferences in a simple, elegant, understandable, and very engaging way. I immediately shared it with my friends and watched as multiple light bulbs went off as they finally "got it."

Of course *I* find personality type fascinating—it's not only provided me with a very satisfying career, but also with daily insights for over thirty years! But like the artist who finds himself standing a little too close to the canvas, for me reading this book was like walking across the room and seeing "type" from another perspective. I was impressed with Renee's ability to employ multiple devices—checklists, spot-on anecdotes, and very funny cartoons—to make some complex ideas not only understandable but immediately useful in real ways.

People who have been immersed in "type" for a long time realize that studying it is a little like peeling an onion. To get to the core, you need to start by first peeling the outermost layers. In *Opposites Attract,* Renee has done an enviable job of helping readers appreciate those outermost layers—people's natural inborn preferences for Extraversion or Introversion, Sensing or Intuition, Thinking or Feeling, and Judging or Perceiving. It is an invitation to begin a journey that provides deep and powerful insights into yourself and the people you care most about.

Knowing your and your mate's individual type preferences is a great start! But no one is *just* a Sensor or Intuitive, a Thinker or Feeler, etc. People are ESTJs . . . INFPs (or one of fourteen other types). And it's the way a person's type preferences *interact* that provides the most powerful insights into who we are, and what we need to be satisfied in a relationship.

If you're interested in taking what you've learned in this book even further, I suggest *Just Your Type: Create the Relationship You've Always Wanted Using the Secrets of Personality Type* (Little Brown, 2000). My co-author Barbara Barron and I set out to learn everything we could about what people of each four-letter type (ISFJ, ENTP, etc.) need to be satisfied, what causes them the greatest conflict, what makes them feel loved or unloved, how they like to be communicated with . . . and *so* much more. And we wanted to know how all this plays out with couples of *every* type combination—136 in all—a daunting task, requiring extensive research.

We administered an on-line survey questionnaire that was filled out by over 2,500 individuals. Then, seven hundred and fifty people completed an extensive, open-ended questionnaire designed to provide even more anecdotal information. Finally, we conducted in-depth interviews with hundreds of couples.

The results demonstrated a strong link between personality type and relationship satisfaction. We looked at twenty-two different aspects of satisfying relationships to determine which were most important to people of different types. Not surprisingly, certain items such as trust, communication, mutual respect, mutual commitment, and fidelity were valued highly by all types. But with some other items, such as shared religious beliefs, financial security, shared interests, similar parenting styles, and having a spiritual connection, there was a great disparity among types. Predictably, when a couple was at odds as to what they valued most as *individuals,* conflict often ensued.

Our research demonstrated clearly just how much type similarities and differences can affect the quality of communication and relationship satisfaction.

In reading *Just Your Type,* you'll first gain an in-depth understanding both of your own and your partner's personality type; how you change over time, your gifts as partners, and what satisfies you in relationships. Once you understand these basics, you can turn to a chapter devoted exclusively to couples of your same type combination (ESTJ with INFP, etc.). Here you learn the joys, the frustrations, and, most important, the tried-and-true strategies that couples very much like you have learned really work!

I'm delighted you've discovered Renee's excellent introduction to personality type, *Opposites Attract.* I hope it has inspired you to want to learn more and I invite you to deepen your understanding by reading in *Just Your Type* which can help you and your partner create the relationship you've always wanted.

—Paul D. Tieger
Just Your Type
Hartford, CT
October 2010

Other books by Paul D. Tieger and Barbara Barron:

- *Do What You Are*

- *Nurture by Nature*

- *The Art of SpeedReading People*

A Brief Description
of the Sixteen
Personality Types

Sensing Judging (SJ) Types: Duty Seekers

SJs are motivated by a need to be useful and of service. They like to stick to the standard ways of doing things and value the traditions, customs, and laws of society.

ESTJ

Outgoing, energetic, and dependable. Efficient, organized, and decisive. Likes administrating and being in charge. Excellent at organizing and deciding policies and procedures. Assertive, outspoken, and direct. Focuses on solving problems. Responsible, hardworking, and goal-oriented. Consistent, pragmatic, and logical.

ISTJ

Reserved, persevering, loyal, and careful. Systematic, organized, and focused on the facts. Hardworking, thorough, and good at follow-through. Down-to-earth, pragmatic, and trustworthy. Honors commitments. Does what is "right" and expects the same of others. Calm and consistent in a crisis.

ESFJ

Enthusiastic, sociable, and engaging. Likes to be needed and appreciated. Personable, sympathetic, and cooperative. Likes being helpful; active in service organizations. Trustworthy, loyal, and responsible. Values harmony and shows love in practical ways.

ISFJ

Conscientious, trustworthy, and cooperative. Loyal, dependable, and self-disciplined. Strong work ethic; completes tasks on time. Excellent memory for details. Quietly friendly, thoughtful, and reserved. Often works behind the scenes helping others. Modest and unassuming. Warm, tactful, and gentle.

Sensing Perceiving (SP) Types: Action Seekers

SPs are motivated by a need for freedom and action. They value and enjoy living in the here and now.

ESTP

Likes risk, challenge, and adventure. Energetic and constantly on the go. Lives life to the fullest. Alert, confident, and persuasive. Can be outrageous, direct, and impulsive. Competent and resourceful. Responds well to crises. Realistic, pragmatic, and matter-of-fact. Skillful negotiator.

ISTP

Prefers action to conversation. Likes adventure and challenge. Does well in a crisis. Enjoys working with tools, machines, and anything requiring hands-on skills. Resourceful, independent, and self-determined. Logical, realistic, and practical. Reserved, detached, curious observer. Storehouse of information and facts.

ESFP

Caring, generous, and cooperative. Enjoys helping others. Friendly, gregarious, energetic, vivacious, and charming. Often the life of the party. Tolerant and accepting of self and others. Has practical common sense. Accentuates the positive. Enjoys new experiences and has zest for life.

ISFP

Gentle, loyal, and compassionate. Appears reserved and unassuming. Quietly does things for others. Patient, accepting, and nonjudgmental. Has a live-and-let-live attitude. Sensitive to conflicts and disagreement. Has little need to dominate or control others.

Intuiting Thinking (NT) Types: Knowledge Seekers

NTs are motivated by a need to understand the world around them. They value competency and the powers of the mind.

ENTJ

Confident leader who likes to be in charge. Decisive and ambitious. Likes intellectual exchange. Ingenious and resourceful in solving complex problems. Innovative, analytical, and logical. Self-determined and independent. Aspires to be the best at whatever he or she does.

ENTP

Outspoken and thrives on challenge and debate. Enthusiastic, charming, gregarious, and witty. Values freedom and independence. Innovative, enterprising, and resourceful. Spontaneous and impulsive. Risk-taker who is alert to all possibilities. Inquisitive and curious.

INTJ

Independent and individualistic. Has great insight and vision. Skilled in creating theories and systems. Drives self and others toward goals and self-improvement. Ingenious and creative problem-solver. Organized, determined, and good at follow-through. Responsible, reserved, and private.

INTP

Analytical and brilliant. Conceptual problem-solver and original thinker. Idiosyncratic and nonconforming. Values precision in thought and language. Notices inconsistencies, contradictions, and logical flaws in others' thinking. Independent, curious, and insightful. Private, aloof, and introspective.

Intuiting Feeling (NF) Types: Ideal Seekers

NFs are motivated by a need to understand themselves and others. They value authenticity and integrity and strive for an ideal world.

ENFJ

Friendly, charming, enthusiastic, and socially active. Persuasive speaker and inspiring, charismatic leader who motivates others. Empathic, warm, helpful, and supportive. Can idealize people and relationships. Responsible, conscientious, and goal-oriented. Diplomatic and good at promoting harmony.

ENFP

Warm-spirited, helpful, accepting, and compassionate. Full of enthusiasm and new ideas. Values freedom and autonomy. Good at communicating and inspiring action. Creative, spontaneous, positive, and fun-loving. Individualistic, insightful, and perceptive.

INFJ

Sensitive, deep, and sometimes mystical. Single-minded regarding personal values and convictions. Has a rich inner life and values personal integrity. Creative, original, and idealistic. Reserved, gentle, and compassionate. Enjoys solitude, yet has a strong need for harmony. Conscientious, determined, and persevering.

INFP

Devoted, compassionate, open-minded, and gentle. Dislikes rules, orders, schedules, and deadlines. Likes learning and being absorbed in own projects. Has passionate convictions and is driven to seek ideals. Sets high standards for self. Idealistic, sensitive, and creative. Can be reserved and contemplative.

Combining the Myers-Briggs Type Indicator Preferences with the Enneagram Types

There are many different systems for studying the human personality. The two that I have found to be the most comprehensive are the MBTI instrument and the Enneagram. I have studied each one separately and discovered that combining the two can offer even greater insight than either one standing alone.

The MBTI instrument looks at our inborn preferences, focuses on our strengths, and encourages self-acceptance and tolerance. The Enneagram looks at how we adapt to the world. It focuses on the habits of mind that limit us and the needs that motivate our behavior. It encourages us to expand our limited view of ourselves and the world and to break through our psychological blocks.

When you understand your own or someone else's MBTI preferences and Enneagram type, it gives you even more insight into a person's underlying motivations. For example, two feeling types have a lot in common, but adding the filter of their Enneagram type can explain some fundamental differences in their motivations. A Feeling Type Four is motivated by the need to understand and express her deepest feelings and discover what is authentic in herself. A Feeling Type Nine is motivated by the need to keep the peace and create a harmonious and comfortable life.

What follows is a simplified explanation of the Enneagram system and a brief description of the nine Enneagram types, followed by an explanation of the eight MBTI preferences and how each preference affects the Enneagram type. If you would like to learn more and read an introductory book on the system, I suggest *The Enneagram Made Easy*.

The Enneagram

The Enneagram is a system of nine personality types whose roots go back many centuries. It is believed to have been taught orally in secret Sufi brotherhoods in the Middle East. The Russian mystic and spiritual teacher Gurdjieff introduced the Enneagram system to Europe in the 1920s, and it arrived in the United States in the late 1960s through Oscar Ichazo. The system is represented by a circle containing a nine-pointed starlike shape. *Ennea* is Greek for the number nine, and *gram* means a drawing or something written.

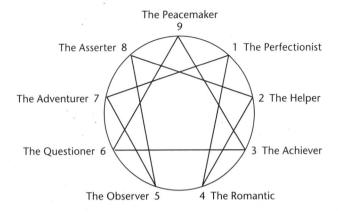

The Peacemaker 9 · The Asserter 8 · The Perfectionist 1 · The Adventurer 7 · The Helper 2 · The Questioner 6 · The Achiever 3 · The Observer 5 · The Romantic 4

The nine personality types in the Enneagram are based on the coping strategies we develop in childhood to deal with the outer world. These strategies may seem to work on one level, but they also limit our view of reality and create habitual ways in which we see and respond to life. The Enneagram looks at the needs that motivate what we do and helps us make sense of our own and others' behavior. We may all relate to some of the qualities of the various Enneagram types. However, each of us has only one core type that represents our underlying motivation. Whatever type we are we remain for life, but we may move up or down the scale of healthy or unhealthy behavior of that particular type.

A Brief Description of the Nine Enneagram Types

One: The Perfectionist

Perfectionists are motivated by the need to live the right way. This includes improving themselves, others, and the world around them. They try to avoid criticism by doing things perfectly. Ones have a strong inner critic or conscience; they live by an internal list of rules and discipline themselves to do what they should do. Healthy Ones are self-disciplined, hardworking, organized, conscientious, and productive. They have high standards and moral principles. Unhealthy

Ones are rigid, inflexible, controlling, self-righteous, overly serious, and hypercritical of themselves and others.

Extraverted Ones are outgoing and talkative. Direct and straightforward, they often impose their high standards on others. Many are leaders.

Introverted Ones are more private, reserved, and self-contained. They concentrate well and are difficult to distract. They tend to direct their high standards toward improving themselves.

Sensing Ones are practical, pragmatic, and detail-oriented. They tend to be more traditional and conservative than intuitive Ones.

Intuitive Ones tend to be innovative, individualistic, and resourceful in solving complex problems and are committed to their inspirations and ideals. They are usually less traditional than sensing Ones.

Thinking Ones are logical and analytical. They are good at making impersonal, objective decisions. They tend to be frank and forthright, critical and controlling. Ones are often Thinkers.

Feeling Ones are often empathic and compassionate, tend to foster harmony, and value helping people. They can be sensitive and fearful of criticism.

Judging Ones are organized, orderly, precise, and efficient. Goal-oriented and decisive, they get things accomplished and can be impatient and frustrated with slow processes. Most Ones are Judgers.

Perceiving Ones are more flexible, adaptable, and spontaneous. A perceiving preference helps balance the One's tendency to be rigid and controlling.

Two: The Helper

Helpers are motivated by the need to be loved, appreciated, and needed. They take pride in their ability to make people feel special and to anticipate and fulfill other people's needs better than anyone else. They appear cheerful, self-sufficient, and confident and are often unaware of their own needs. Healthy Twos are warm, generous, empathic, enthusiastic, and nurturing. They relate easily to people, enjoy giving to others, and are capable of unconditional love. Unhealthy Twos are manipulative, clingy, indirect, possessive, martyrlike, and preoccupied with gaining approval.

Extraverted Twos are enthusiastic, expressive, and effusive and relate with warmth and affection to many people. They are often outgoing, friendly, and talkative. Most Twos are extraverted.

More reserved, introverted Twos are quietly helpful behind the scenes.

Sensing Twos show their love and caring in practical ways by doing things for others. Often traditional and conservative, they are concerned about being socially appropriate.

Intuitive Twos are often insightful, inspiring, and imaginative. They are full of enthusiasm and new ideas for helping, potentiating, and persuading others. They are less traditional than sensing Twos.

Thinking Twos are uncommon. Being objective, logical, analytical, and emotionally detached are traits that are foreign to the Two personality type.

Feeling Twos are nurturing, warm, empathic, and supportive. They are cooperative and value harmony. Almost all Twos are feeling types.

Judging Twos tend to be orderly, organized, and always capable of getting things done. They are usually more controlling than perceiving Twos.

Perceiving Twos tend to be adaptable and spontaneous and can have difficulty with completion and follow-through. They value freedom and autonomy and can be overwhelmed by details.

Three: The Achiever

Achievers are motivated by the need to be productive, efficient, admired, and successful at whatever they do. Avoiding failure is very important to them. Life is a series of tasks and goals to be completed, and they keep pushing themselves to achieve more. They are often disconnected from their deeper feelings and may lose an inner sense of themselves. Healthy Threes are energetic, charming, optimistic, confident, self-assured, and competent. They make good leaders who motivate others to live up to their potential. Unhealthy Threes are vain, overly competitive, deceitful, superficial, narcissistic, opportunistic, and prone to putting on facades to impress people.

Extraverted Threes are outgoing, sociable, and friendly. Being energetic, enthusiastic, and charming, they are often good communicators. They like to be in the limelight and can be inspiring and persuasive leaders. Extraverted Threes are common.

Introverted Threes are more reserved and self-contained and less apt to be at the center of public attention. They are less common than extraverted Threes.

Sensing Threes are realistic, practical, and pragmatic. Their attention is focused on the here and now. They're usually more traditional than Intuitive Threes.

Intuitive Threes are innovative, ingenious, and visionary in inventing new ways of doing things and meeting their goals.

Thinking Threes are analytical, objective, rational, and logical. They are resourceful in solving challenging problems and often become heads of organizations. Direct, straightforward, and outspoken, they can be impatient, controlling, and tough-minded.

Feeling Threes are empathetic and supportive and value harmony and cooperation. They're highly communicative—especially those who are extraverted—and good at inspiring and persuading others. They are often leaders and are more likely to be women than men.

Judging Threes are organized, efficient, decisive, and determined as they work to reach their goals. Most Threes are judging types.

Perceiving Threes are more spontaneous and adaptable. They like variety and change, risk and challenge, and resist anything that limits or traps them. They are less common than judging Threes.

Four: The Romantic

Romantics are motivated by the need to understand and express their deepest feelings and to discover what is authentic in themselves. They want to feel special and unique and avoid being seen as ordinary. Their attention is focused on whatever is missing, distant, and idealized. Healthy Fours are imaginative, sensitive, intuitive, creative, and compassionate. They are introspective, self-aware, and in touch with the hidden depths of human nature. Unhealthy Fours are self-absorbed, hypersensitive, impractical, self-loathing, moody, depressed, and envious of those who seem more fulfilled than they are.

Extraverted Fours are verbally expressive, often dramatic, and more outgoing than Fours tend to be. Extraversion balances the Four's inward tendencies.

Introverted Fours are more reserved or withdrawn and have a quiet, low-key presence. Most Fours are introverted.

Sensing Fours are more practical, down-to-earth, and present in here-and-now reality than intuitive Fours. Sensing helps balance the Four's tendency to live in the imagination and fantasy. They are less common than intuitive Fours.

Intuitive Fours are imaginative, insightful, and idealistic and have passionate convictions. They are often complex, individualistic, and intense. Most Fours are Intuitives.

Thinking Fours are uncommon. Being objective, analytical, rational, and emotionally detached are traits that do not fit the Four personality type.

Feeling Fours are warmhearted, compassionate, and empathic. They can be emotionally sensitive and moody. Most Fours are feeling types.

Judging Fours are organized, orderly, and persevering in getting things done. This preference helps balance the Four's tendency to put off doing things until they're in the right mood.

Perceiving Fours are more impulsive, spontaneous, and adaptable. They can delay putting plans and goals into action.

Five: The Observer

Observers are motivated by the need to gain knowledge and to be independent and self-sufficient. They observe life from a distance, guard their privacy and space, and avoid being engulfed by others. They feel more safe and in control when thinking and analyzing than when in their feelings. They are individualistic and not influenced by social pressure or material possessions. Healthy Fives are objective, focused, calm, perceptive, insightful, and curious. They have ingenious insight. Unhealthy Fives are intellectually arrogant, withholding, controlled, cynical, negative, standoffish, and stingy.

Extraverted Fives are more direct and outspoken, and less private and reserved, than Fives tend to be. This preference helps these Fives be more active and participatory in life rather than observing from the sidelines. Extraverted Fives are not common.

Introverted Fives are reserved, calm, and self-contained, as Fives tend to be. They are soft-spoken and have a quiet, knowing presence.

Sensing Fives are practical, pragmatic, and matter-of-fact. Technically oriented, they often enjoy working with tools and machines.

Intuitive Fives are introspective, insightful, and ingenious problem-solvers. Scholarly and visionary, they have strong conceptual strengths and are often innovators in the field of ideas. Most Fives are Intuitive types.

Thinking Fives are logical, analytical, and theoretical problem-solvers. They are objective, cool, dispassionate, and impersonal. Most Fives are thinking types.

Feeling Fives are less common. The exceptions tend to be more gentle, tactful, tuned-in, and sensitive to people. They are often moody and melancholy, aware of their inner world, and sensitive to criticism. They're more likely to be women than men.

Judging Fives tend to be organized, follow through on their commitments and goals, and are intent on seeing their ideas developed and applied. This preference helps balance the Five's tendency to make constant preparations but not take action. Judging Fives can be controlling and demanding of themselves and others.

Perceiving Fives are less focused on completion and putting their ideas out into the world. They can get sidetracked by possibilities.

Six: The Questioner

Questioners are motivated by the need to feel secure and in control and to have safety and predictability. Feeling a sense of belonging and finding someone trustworthy to depend on are important goals to them. Tried-and-tested laws, norms, or rules help them feel safe. Sixes often identify with a person, group, or cause on which they depend for protection. Sixes are careful and cautious about life's dangers and potential attacks. Sixes have an ambivalent relationship to authority. They often distrust and are suspicious of it and are not comfortable being seen as the authority themselves. Some Sixes are phobic and withdraw to protect themselves, whereas others are counterphobic and confront fearful situations head-on, even seeking them out. Healthy Sixes are trustworthy, responsible, alert, insightful, loyal, compassionate, and sympathetic to underdog causes. Unhealthy Sixes are hypervigilant, indecisive, defensive, testy, self-defeating, paranoid, and preoccupied with worst-case scenarios.

Extraverted Sixes are outgoing, social, and talkative. They often value being a group member.

Introverted Sixes are more reserved, quiet, and private.

Sensing Sixes are practical and pragmatic. Dutiful and dependable, they tend to be more traditional than intuitive Sixes.

Intuitive Sixes are often visionary, insightful, and innovative, and they are ingenious problem-solvers.

Thinking Sixes are objective, logical, and analytical. They thrive on challenge and debate and are more antiauthoritarian and counterphobic than feeling Sixes.

Feeling Sixes are caring, concerned, and compassionate. Loyal and supportive, they tend to be more dependent and phobic than thinking Sixes.

Judging Sixes are responsible, hardworking, organized, and efficient and are good at completing tasks.

Perceiving Sixes are adaptable, spontaneous, and impulsive. They are less rule-bound and structured than judging Sixes.

Seven: The Adventurer

Adventurers are motivated by the need to be happy and to stay busy by keeping their options open and constantly making plans for new experiences. They view life as a fun-filled adventure, yet they also want to contribute to the world. Constant seekers of excitement, Sevens try to avoid boredom, suffering, painful emotions, and the everyday drudgeries of life. Healthy Sevens are optimistic, enthusiastic, spontaneous, idealistic, curious, generous, and often multitalented. They uplift and enliven others and are fun to be around. Unhealthy Sevens are self-centered, self-indulgent, insensitive, narcissistic, hyperactive, and undisciplined, and they have problems with completion and long-term commitments.

Extraverted Sevens are energetic, exuberant, and enthusiastic. Most are outgoing, gregarious, charming, and charismatic. Dynamic and persuasive, they are highly verbal and are good at dealing with the public. Most Sevens are extraverted.

Introverted Sevens are more reserved and private. This preference helps Sevens balance the desire to be so externally focused. Introverted Sevens are less common.

Sensing Sevens are realistic, practical, pragmatic, and present in the here and now. Action-oriented, they respond well to crisis.

Intuitive Sevens are innovative and insightful and focused on future possibilities. They are imaginative and ingenious in inventing new ways of doing and seeing things.

Thinking Sevens are logical, objective, analytical, and resourceful in solving challenging problems. Often direct and outspoken, they thrive on challenge and debate. They can be insensitive to others.

Feeling Sevens are helpful, supportive, sympathetic, and compassionate. This preference helps balance the Seven's tendency to be insensitive and self-centered.

Judging Sevens tend to be more organized and decisive and are good at follow-through. They are less prone to being impulsive. This preference helps Sevens stay on task.

Perceiving Sevens like variety and change and are resistant to anything that limits, traps, or bores them. They can have difficulty seeing projects through to completion. They are good at improvising and thinking on their feet. Most Sevens are perceiving types.

Eight: The Asserter

Asserters are motivated by the need to feel powerful and self-reliant and to have control over their lives. They avoid being weak, vulnerable, controlled by others, or taken advantage of. Being respected for their strength is more important to them than being liked. They are earthy and lusty, and they go after whatever they want. They tend to milk enjoyment out of life. They are natural leaders who want to make an impact on the world. Healthy Eights are confident, direct, decisive, courageous, and protective of their loved ones. Unhealthy Eights are aggressive, confrontational, domineering, self-centered, insensitive, and prone to excess.

Extraverted Eights are outgoing, energetic, and exuberant. They like responsibility, control, and being in charge. Often outspoken, strong, and forceful, they can be powerful leaders. Extraverted Eights are common.

Introverted Eights are private and reserved and less likely to be in the public eye. They can be quietly controlling.

Sensing Eights are practical, pragmatic, down-to-earth, and imbued with common sense. They are more conservative and rule-bound than intuitive Eights.

Intuitive Eights tend to be visionary and oriented to future possibilities. Often innovative leaders, they are less traditional than sensing Eights.

Thinking Eights are direct, outspoken, and often in charge. They can be argumentative, opinionated, confrontational, and challenging. Eights tend to be thinking types, especially male Eights.

Feeling Eights are warmhearted, helpful, and supportive. They are less forceful and controlling than thinking Eights, unless pushed or treated unfairly, and they are more aware of how their behavior affects others. Feeling helps balance the Eight's tendency to be insensitive to others. These Eights are more likely to be women than men.

Judging Eights are organized, efficient, and decisive. Persevering and goal-oriented, they like responsibility, control, and being in charge. Most Eights are judging types.

Perceiving Eights are spontaneous and impulsive and sometimes reckless. They are less likely to be controlling than judging Eights.

Nine: The Peacemaker

Peacemakers are motivated by a need to keep the peace and create a harmonious and comfortable life. They disregard their own needs and priorities to accommodate others and avoid conflict. They are disconnected from their own emotions, especially their anger. They like to merge with others and with their environment, and they gain their sense of self through these connections. Healthy Nines are adaptable, compassionate, easygoing, supportive, patient, and nonjudgmental; they go with the flow. Unhealthy Nines are indecisive, spaced-out, apathetic, undisciplined, unassertive, passive-aggressive, and stubborn.

Extraverted Nines are outgoing, friendly, and talkative. They are more open to sharing their thoughts and feelings than introverted Nines.

Introverted Nines are reserved and quietly friendly. Modest, gentle, and unassuming, they often prefer staying in the background, behind the scenes. Nines are often Introverts.

Sensing Nines are practical, down-to-earth, and grounded in present reality. They tend to be more traditional and conservative than intuitive Nines.

Intuitive Nines are idealistic and imaginative and interested in the world of ideas and possibilities. Their attention is focused on what *might* be or what *could* be, not on what *is*. Staying grounded in the present can be challenging. They are usually less traditional than sensing Nines.

Thinking Nines are analytical and objective. They are more apt to be direct and outspoken and can be strong-willed and stubborn. A preference for thinking mitigates the Nine's tendency to be conflict-avoidant.

Feeling Nines are gentle, empathetic, sensitive, and compassionate. Accommodating, accepting, and agreeable unless crossed, they value harmony. It is common for Nines to be feeling types.

Judging Nines tend to be orderly, organized, decisive, and productive. Nines with this preference are less likely to procrastinate and put things off to the last minute.

Perceiving Nines tend to be easygoing, adaptable, and spontaneous. They have a live-and-let-live, go-with-the-flow mentality. They can have difficulty with completion and follow-through. It is common for Nines to be perceiving types.

Recommended Resources

Baron, Renee. *What Type Am I?* (Penguin, 2004).

Baron, Renee, and Elizabeth Wagele. *The Enneagram Made Easy* (Harper-Collins, 1994).

———. *Are You My Type, Am I Yours?* (HarperCollins, 1995).

Hirsh, Sandra K., and Jane A. G. Kise. *Soul Types: Matching Your Personality and Spiritual Path* (Hyperion, 1998).

Hirsh, Sandra K., and Jean M. Kummerow. *LIFETypes: Understand Yourself and Make the Most of Who You Are* (Warner Books, 1989).

Kroeger, Otto, and Janet Thuesen. *Type Talk* (Delacorte Press, 1998).

———. *Type Talk at Work* (Dell, 2002).

Laney, Marti Olsen. *The Introvert Advantage: How to Thrive in an Extrovert World* (Workman Publishing, 2002).

Myers, Isabel Briggs, and Peter B. Myers. *Gifts Differing: Understanding Personality Type* (CPP, 1980).

Pearman, Roger R., and Sarah C. Albritton. *I'm Not Crazy, I'm Just Not You: The Real Meaning of the 16 Personality Types* (Davies-Black, 1997).

Penley, Janet P., and Diane Eble. *MotherStyles: Using Personality Type to Discover Your Parenting Strengths* (Da Capo Press, 2006).

Tieger, Paul D., and Barbara Barron. *Nurture by Nature: How to Raise Happy, Healthy, Responsible Children Through the Insights of Personality Type* (Little, Brown & Co., 1997).

———. *Just Your Type: Create the Relationship You've Always Wanted Using the Secrets of Personality Type* (Little, Brown & Co., 2000).

———. *Do What You Are: Discover the Perfect Career for You Through the Secrets of Personality Type* (Little, Brown & Co., 2007).

Acknowledgments

Thanks to . . .

Cindy DiTiberio, my editor at HarperOne, for her support and many wise suggestions. Her interest in the MBTI, which she was steeped in from a young age by her father, an MBTI teacher and enthusiast, made her a sensitive and thoughtful collaborator for this project.

Autumn Stephens, my freelance editor, whose clarity, intelligence, and humor made every sentence come to life. When I got an edited chapter back, I was always amazed at how it read. She might have gotten tired of hearing the praise. (She said she didn't.) I am grateful for her presence in my life. To contact Autumn: astephens@earthlink.net.

Anne Gibbons, my illustrator, who was a delight to work with. The minute I saw her work, I knew I wanted to hire her. Somehow, she intuited exactly how I would have drawn each cartoon—if, that is, I could draw. To contact Anne: ag@annegibbons.com.

Luna Baron, my daughter, who has edited many of my books. She provided much-needed support in launching this project and helped me gain clarity as I worked to give shape to my ideas. Throughout this and other projects, our insightful discussions about the Enneagram and MBTI have resulted in some darn funny cartoons as well as further insight into personality types.

Sandra Delay, my good friend, who kindly made herself available in the final weeks of manuscript creation to help finalize my decisions. As always, she was a wonderful companion on the journey toward deeper understanding of the Enneagram and MBTI personality types.

And finally, thanks to you, my readers, for your continued interest in my work, and for providing a forum for my teaching about personality type. I am deeply appreciative.